# BLIND TRUST IN DOCTORS AND WHY ITS KILLING YOU

# +

# BENEFITS OF PLANT BASED MEDICINE

# BLIND TRUST IN DOCTORS AND WHY ITS KILLING YOU

*Medical Myths, lies and Misconceptions you've blindly believed about health fitness and weight loss. A patient's guide to preventative medicine and why it could save your life.*

**Howard Mason**

# © Copyright 2019 - All rights reserved.

The content contained within this book may not be reproduced, duplicated or transmitted without direct written permission from the author or the publisher.

Under no circumstances will any blame or legal responsibility be held against the publisher, or author, for any damages, reparation, or monetary loss due to the information contained within this book, either directly or indirectly.

Legal Notice:

This book is copyright protected. It is only for personal use. You cannot amend, distribute, sell, use, quote or paraphrase any part, or the content within this book, without the consent of the author or publisher.

Disclaimer Notice:

Please note the information contained within this document is for educational and entertainment purposes only. All effort has been executed to present accurate, up to date, reliable, complete information. No warranties of any kind are declared or implied. Readers acknowledge that the author is not engaging in the rendering of legal, financial, medical or professional advice. The content within this book has been derived from various sources. Please consult a licensed professional before attempting any techniques outlined in this book.

By reading this document, the reader agrees that under no circumstances is the author responsible for any losses, direct or indirect, that are incurred as a result of the use of information contained within this document, including, but not limited to, errors, omissions, or inaccuracies.

# Table Of Contents

**Introduction** ................................................................. 7
**Chapter 1: Can You Trust Your Doctor's Advice?** ..... 10
  Your Doctor is Only Human................................................ 10
    The Business of Medicine ................................................12
    What is Prescribed for You and What is Good for
    You .......................................................................................14
**Chapter 2: Pharmaceutical Corruption** .................... 16
  Big Pharma ..............................................................................16
    We are Clients, not Patients .............................................18
  The Control .............................................................................19
    Murdered by Medication ...................................................21
  FDA Recalls ............................................................................ 24
**Chapter 3: Fat and Weight Loss** ............................... 27
  The Truth About Diets and Weight Loss .......................... 28
    Lies About Weight Loss .................................................... 33
**Chapter 4: Foods Your Body Needs and the
Pyramid of Lies** ........................................................... 38
  What You Should Be Eating ..................................................41
**Chapter 5: The Cardio Myth: Exercise Smart** ......... 45
  The Big Lies ............................................................................ 45
    The Biggest Lies ................................................................ 50
**Chapter 6: The Cholesterol Myth** ............................ 56
  The Bad Cholesterol - LDL ....................................................57
  The Good Cholesterol – HDL ................................................57
  Triglycerides ........................................................................... 58
  What You Need to Know About Cholesterol ..................... 58
  Other Causes of Heart Disease ........................................... 59
  Controlling Your Cholesterol Levels ....................................61
    Foods that Lower LDL Levels and Raise HDL Levels.... 62
**Chapter 7: Stop Counting Calories** ......................... 66
  The Calorie Myth ................................................................... 66
    The Importance of Quality over Quantity ..................... 68

Exercise Smart .................................................................. 70
Eating Smart .................................................................... 73
**Chapter 8: Eating to Prevent Cancer ........................ 75**
Red Meat and Processed Meat ....................................... 75
Cancer Causing Foods ..................................................... 77
Cancer Preventing Foods ................................................ 83
Tips for Further Cancer Prevention ............................... 88
**Chapter 9: Carbs Don't Fuel Your Brain ................. 90**
How Does the Brain Work? ............................................. 91
The Source of Glucose ..................................................... 92
Ketone Bodies .................................................................. 93
Carbohydrates versus Fat and Protein ........................... 94
**Chapter 10: Viruses and Antibiotics ....................... 96**
What are Antibiotics? ...................................................... 96
Why Can't Antibiotics Kill Viruses? ............................... 97
Antibiotic Resistance and Resistant Bacteria ................ 98
Don't Take Them if You Don't Need Them ................... 100
Curing Viral and Bacterial Infections Correctly ............. 101
**Conclusion ................................................................ 103**
**References ................................................................ 106**

# Introduction

Let me set the scene for you:

You're sitting in a doctor's office awaiting your turn to go in and see him. This is the third time you've been here with the same problem. The last time you were here he prescribed you some expensive drugs and assured you that you'd feel better once you started taking them. You did everything the doctor told you to. You even got those expensive drugs, but now you're back. Why? Because you still aren't feeling better and it's all the doctors fault. He must have prescribed you the wrong medicine, right? Or maybe he was wrong about what illness you have. Or maybe it's both.

We've all been in this situation or one similar to it at some point. We trust our doctors and the people whose job it is to protect us and guard our health. Why shouldn't we trust them? After all, they get paid to make sure we're healthy.

That is the exact reason why we cannot trust them.

The medical industry and everyone involved in it makes money off of our health. If we were to become healthy, we wouldn't need them anymore and then they would stop making money. They rely on the public's illness and inability to get better on thier own. Without us they would be out of a job. So no, we cannot trust our doctor or anyone in the medical, food, or weight-loss and diet industries. There are some good doctors out there, but the majority of them are just looking out for themselves at the end of the day and we can't and shouldn't trust them with our lives.

This is one of the biggest problems we have to deal with today.

Who do we trust with our bodies, health, and lives? The only person we can fully trust is ourselves. The medical industry is just out to make money and they can't make money off of the healthy. The food industry is just a part of the medical industry and they're out for the same thing. They control what we think is okay to eat so we spend money on the things they want us to buy. The weight-loss and diet industries are no better. They create new and improved diets for people to try with little to no scientific research to back what they're saying. Only one word screams loud enough in their ears for them to hear: profit. Since everyone out there is just out to make as much profit as possible, the only person you can trust is yourself.

It's up to you to take care of your own body and your own health. This isn't just something you can do, of course. Medical professions study for years to be able to tell you what's wrong with you and they still get it wrong sometimes. What we can do is listen to what these people have to tell us but then take every single word through a strainer. Use this strainer as a way to find out the truth. Let all the lies seep through until only the absolute truth remains.

These days we have a lot of information that is readily available to us. All we have to do is type out our question and search through all the answers until enough of them match up and ring out as true. That is how we can combat the pool of lies these industries have us swimming in.

We can ask them questions, but sometimes we forget that we can. I was once like that, but one day I decided that what they were telling me wasn't good enough. I wanted to know more, so I started asking questions. Eventually I gave them questions that they couldn't even answer, so I had to go find the answers myself. I've spent years learning all that I can about the body and how it works. I've learnt all the ways we can keep our bodies healthy. I found out about all the 'facts' that the doctors were telling me and realized that they weren't facts but myths. The world of health is filled with myths. That was the hard part, but I found them all.

Once you get through all the myths and the lies, you start to see the truth. I managed to find the truth and with it I have changed my life for the better. I am healthy, fit, and this is all without the help of diet and medical companies. You can do it, too. I vow to show you through all the myths and lead you on the path to the cold, hard truth. There will be bumps and stops along the road but eventually I will help you free yourself from the money grabbing clutches of the big industries.

I can not only point out the myths and lies they use to control you. I can also show you the only truth you will ever need to know. When we're finished you'll be healthy, fit, and have a better lifestyle, one that is worth living to its fullest. This is my promise to you.

I urge you now to take the first step on your journey to the truth. The longer you wait, the more your body and mind will be poisoned. The best time to start is now. Don't put it off until you're feeling better or until you don't have anything on your plate. If you want to improve your lifestyle and become less dependent on your doctors, then this is the best place to start.

Take my hand and let's get going on this long and hard journey. Through all the mistakes, trials, and errors you will see that it is all worth it. You will be rewarded if you take action and take charge. Your life and your future belong to you and only you. Why should you not take complete control over them?

# Chapter 1:
# Can You Trust Your Doctor's Advice?

We all want to trust our doctors and why shouldn't we expect that we can? Doctors spend several years in medical school training and learning everything they know, but that doesn't mean they know everything. They especially don't know everything that is good for you. I would like to tell you that you can trust your doctor. In fact, in most cases you can. They do know more about what is going on inside your body and how to fix certain problems you may be suffering from. However, the problem comes in the information they have but don't want to share or the information that is out there that they don't want to acknowledge.

## Your Doctor is Only Human

Humans aren't perfect, and anyone who believes differently is kidding themselves. Doctors are only human and that means that they aren't perfect either. People make mistakes, and that includes the so called 'experts' in their fields. Anyone can make a mistake. Your accountant could make a mistake, your plumber could mess up, and in the case of your doctor, when they make a mistake it can be fatal. These are the extreme cases, though.

There are plenty of stories about the doctors who have messed up or made a mistake. Some of these mistakes had huge consequences; others were minor. Still, you wouldn't want to entrust your life to someone who can easily make a mistake and put you in danger. We've all heard a story or two of how a doctor will tell their patient they're good and healthy only to see them end up in the hospital or back at the doctor's office not long afterwards.

I know a story myself of a woman who wasn't feeling very well. She went to the doctor, a man she had been trusting for years with her own and her children's lives. Her doctor said that she had the flu and it was nothing to worry about. A month later, she still wasn't well and was told she had cancer.

There's another story of a doctor who claimed one of his patient's eyes was diseased. Both the patient's eyes were perfectly fine, however the horror story comes in when the doctor goes ahead and operates on the wrong eye. There are a number of stories where doctors have made a mistake or messed up. This can be expected from any expert in their field.

Doctors have also made the opposite mistake by diagnosing their patients with a deadly disease when, in fact, one was not present. We all hope that if we do have a disease that can kill us our doctors will be able to catch it in time. Something we don't expect is for our doctors to tell us we're dying when we still have quite a lot of years ahead of us. These kinds of mistakes can lead people to live their life in fear, even after hearing that the diagnosis is incorrect, and it can cost a lot of money. Remember what I said earlier: all doctors are human, and to err is human.

Don't freak out or get scared now. Your doctor can be right and useful in some cases and you shouldn't throw their advice out altogether. What you should do is not give them any blind, unwavering faith. Take what your doctor says to you under consideration, but don't stop there. When it's your life on the line, you should always get as much involved as you can.

These days we have so much information available to us and it is more easily accessible than it has ever been. The internet is a treasure trove of information. That being said, you also shouldn't believe everything you hear or read on the Internet. There are some horror stories of people Googling their symptoms and ending up with the most extreme results. If you're going to do your research, then make sure you do it right. Remember that your doctor is only human, and so are you. Being a medical profession is hard, however that doesn't excuse the doctors from putting their patient's life in danger without knowing all the facts or while still ignoring some of the facts they do have.

After learning all of this, you can't put full blame on your doctor. They aren't the only ones in the industry. That's what the medical world has become; just another business industry.

## *The Business of Medicine*

Earlier, I mentioned something about how someone could end up spending a lot of money when it was unnecessary. This is another problem we can find within the medical world. The world of medicine has just become another part of the business world. We can't blame the doctors for what they do. They do what anyone else does. They look out for themselves. After all, this is their livelihood and where they make the money they live on. We all want to look out for ourselves and the people we love at the end of the day. However, that doesn't excuse every action a doctor makes. They are still put in a position where people's lives are in their hands and there is a certain level of trust that needs to be held between them. The big medical pharmacies like to squeeze their way in between the doctors and their patients.

There are many medicines out there that a doctor will prescribe that are overly expensive and are used to treat the same symptoms that an even cheaper over the counter drug can treat. Medicine companies are more interested in getting you to spend your money than they are in making sure you're actually getting the medication you need. Pharmaceutical companies are million dollar businesses. It is a highly profitable industry and the people who work in the industry know this. In the end, they are no better than the stock brokers that convince you to buy high knowing very well that there is a high chance you'll lose your money.

To prove my point, we don't have to look any further than a pain medication called Vioxx. For years patients were taking this painkiller after being assured by their doctors that it would help and it was safe. After taking this medication for years to patients learned of the heart problems it causes as a side-effect. Only after suffering heart attacks because of taking the painkiller, Vioxx, did the patients start to look for who was responsible. Of course there were court cases, and punishment was handed out in the sum of some pretty hefty fines.

It was proven that the drug company that made and sold the drug knew of the effects and blatantly disregarded it and their patients. Although it is the big drug companies that should be punished, the doctors shouldn't be let off that easily. Some people found out about the heart problems that Vioxx could cause and they were not medical professionals. They learned about the effects and stopped taking the drug long before anyone else, including doctors, knew about it. What I'm trying to say is that if these doctors actually cared enough, then they would have found out about the effects. If someone who is not a medical professional can learn about the effects of a drug, then a doctor should be able to see those effects long before they prescribe the drug to their patients.

Doctors don't do that. At least, not all of them do. They like to hide behind what the big medicine companies have told them. They also place their blind faith in what they are told. We need to make sure we do not do the same.

This is not an attempt to bash doctors or medical professions and make you untrustworthy of them forever. This is just me asking you to open your eyes and see what is in front of you. You wouldn't fully trust your money with someone else. You wouldn't trust your children with someone you don't know. Don't fully trust your life and your health to a doctor.

## What is Prescribed for You and What is Good for You

These two things are not always the same. The doctor may say he knows what you need to feel better and he'll prescribe you some medication that should help. However, when they are writing that prescription, they're mostly thinking about what they think is wrong with you and the money you're going to spend on the drugs. They aren't thinking about how the drug may affect you in other areas.

Maybe you're trying to lose weight and the doctor prescribes you a drug that increases your cravings and appetite. Perhaps you have bad skin and the drug you've been prescribed can make your skin even worse. This has happened to me before.

I was on a diet and on my way to losing weight when my doctor gave me some medication that increased my cravings. The medication was working for my illness but at the same time I was eating uncontrollably and gaining weight like there was no tomorrow. Not long after realizing that it was the medication that caused my cravings, I also learned that there was another drug with the same effects as the one I was taking. This drug wasn't that much cheaper than the one I was taking but it could have gotten the job done without increasing my cravings and making me gain weight. My point here is that a doctor will prescribe you the correct medication to help you with whatever problem you are having, but that doesn't mean that it's all around good for you.

It's always good to ask your doctor questions about the medication they want you to take. Up to 96% of patients in the

U.S. don't ask questions about their medication. This is an astounding number of people who are blindly taking medication because they just trust that their doctor knows what they're doing. You have a right to ask as many questions as you want. It's your body and your health on the line.

Basically, don't be afraid to ask questions. Don't just ask your doctor more about the medication he is prescribing you, ask your pharmacist as well. The truth is that the pharmacist has probably been studying drugs longer than the doctor has so ask both of them all the questions you want.

When your doctor wants you to take a medication, ask him and your pharmacist for all of the possible side-effects the medication may have. Ask them if there is another cheaper option available or an option that has fewer side-effects. Once you've asked your questions and gotten your answers, don't stop there. Do your own research. Find out everything there is to find out then cross check that information with what your doctor is telling you to see if they match.

It's usually a good idea to listen to what your doctor tells you and to follow their advice. However, that doesn't mean you have to blindly trust in them. Without even going into detail, or mentioning any horror stories, I can tell you that a doctor simply won't tell you everything. They won't tell you about the expected side-effects of a medication unless you ask them. They won't tell you about those cheaper over the counter options that will give you the same results. It's better for them if you choose the more expensive prescription drugs. Remember that your doctor is just like you and me. They're only human and they're looking out for themselves and their families. That's what we all do. Don't let this put you off doctors completely because at the end of the day we do need them. What we don't need is to put all of our trust and faith in them, as if they are perfect and won't make a mistake.

# Chapter 2: Pharmaceutical Corruption

Let's talk about the medical industry and Big Pharma. These are the people who are trusted with our health. We all trust the medical industry with our lives. but should we? We are led to believe that they are here to heal us and that they actually care about our health. This, however, is not true. We talked about doctors earlier and how we cannot trust them blindly. Even if there are some good doctors out there that actually care about their patient's well-being, those few doctors are powerless against the Big Pharmaceutical companies.

These companies own the entirety of the medical world, including everything and everyone that has anything to do with it. This wouldn't be that much of a problem if they weren't all riddled with corruption. For the pharmaceutical companies it's not about making people feel better, or about finding a cure for a disease. For them it's all about the profit. They don't care to cure a disease or heal the people because the moment someone stops needing their medicine, then they stop making money. So, let's talk about how Big Pharma are killing us instead of healing us. Let's talk about how they own and control every part of the medical industry.

## Big Pharma

Although Big Pharma has a tight grip on the medical industry, they are still a new idea. The big pharmaceutical companies have been in their position of power for a short amount of time. Still, in this time they have become guilty of many unforgivable crimes, and that is including murder. The way Big Pharma is designed means that a small number of people or families are able to own all of it. I hope this sounds as ridiculous to you as it does to me. A small number of families are the shareholders of the biggest contributors to our medical industry. This small number of families is the owner of the majority of the world. That screams corruption.

John D. Rockefeller is the prime founder of the industry, a man who made the majority of his money through his Standard Oil Company. Rockefeller was quoted once saying that 'competition is a sin,' so he was responsible for removing all of the competition that the medical industry had to offer him. He used his petrochemical products to create chemicals which were later sold as medicine, and this was just the start of his mission to control and corrupt the medical world.

Rockefeller offered extremely large grants to universities so he could control the medical schools and their publications. This was just the start of the corruption. Every natural remedy or product is outlawed or patented to further their control and power over the industry. They control every medicine that is released to the public and this is the way they generate the most profit possible.

Rockefeller has already been found guilty of corruption, racketeering, and illegal business practices by the Supreme Court of the U.S. This does not stop him from channeling huge amounts of profit into the hands of the few shareholders. That's what matters to them: profits.

They call the shots and they own the world. Proof of this can be found in the lobbyist nature of the medical industry. They spend a lot of money influencing the government to make sure that the right laws are pushed forward so that their profit can be maximized. The medical industry once spent close to $240 million on lobbying. This is how much money they have to give in order to ensure that they remain in control. They spend about $56 billion dollars a year on pharmaceutical marketing in the U.S. If you think about how much money they spend on this and other ridiculous things a year, then you can see for yourself exactly how much profit they make in order to keep spending like this.

### *We are Clients, not Patients*

With the big pharmaceutical companies running on their need for money and profit, it's not hard to see how we have ceased to be patients. We are no longer seen as the sick and the dying. We are seen as clients with pockets filled with money. It makes much more sense for them to treat a disease rather than cure it. The moment someone is cured of their disease is the moment they stop giving their money to the Big Pharma. First and foremost, the reason for the industry is to generate as much profit as possible. They can achieve this through expensive pills and procedures. This is why they suppresses natural remedies or cheaper, over the counter solutions. These natural remedies and cost effective cures make no money for the industry, which makes them useless.

We know that these natural remedies work because there are tests and studies that prove it. Not to mention that these remedies are all that were available to our ancestors who survived many diseases and illnesses. However, this knowledge is kept suppressed and hidden from the public. If we were ever to find out about these cheaper, more natural options, the medical industry would lose most of its clients and profit.

It's in Big Pharma's best interest to keep us as ignorant and dependent on them as possible. That is their goal. They keep us trusting and keep us spending our money on them. That's why when you go to the pharmacist all you will find are endless shelves filled with expensive drugs and you never just need one of them. You will always need more. The drugs are designed to treat one symptom of the disease so you are forced to buy multiple medicines to treat all of your symptoms. That is how much the medical industry has fallen.

## The Control

Big Pharma is in full control of medication. They control the research, development, and creation of all medication that reaches the market. The medical industry owns almost everything. Through corruption they control the medical universities which means that most of the doctors that those universities teach belong to Big Pharma. They control the publication of medical journals and research so that anything they don't want the public to see will never get published.

A former editor of the New England Journal of Medicine said, "The medical profession is being bought by the pharmaceutical industry, not only in terms of practice of medicine, but also in terms of teaching and research."

The universities, researchers, and physicians are allowing themselves to be bought and paid for by Big Pharma. The most important journals in the medical world are also corrupt, a truth that editors slowly found out over the decades of working for them.

A big step in controlling the medical industry involves the publication of medical research, or should I say the 'selective publication.' Richard Horton, an editor of the Lancet, said, "Much of the scientific literature, perhaps half, may simply be untrue."

The medical industry controls what is published so they can control what the people believe about certain medications and drugs. The research itself is paid for by the pharmaceutical companies and they almost always have positive results. Does that not sound suspicious? Trials run by the medical industry have a 70 percent chance of their research showing a positive result. They are 70 percent more likely to have a positive result than research that is government funded. Let's think about that. The numbers just don't make sense.

Negative trials are research projects on a certain drug that show that the drug had no benefit. Negative trials are the ones being suppressed. That's why the positive trial rate is so high, because more of the positives are being published while the negatives are being swept under the rug. The evidence lies in the publication of studies for antidepressants. Of the favorable studies found, 36 out of 37 of them were published. The studies that weren't favorable to the antidepressants were not so lucky, as only 3 out of 36 were published. With these numbers, it shows that 94 percent of studies will find drugs favorable. However, in truth, only 51 percent of the studies were positive.

The company Sanofi completed 92 studies in 2008. Only 14 of them were published! That is because the people in control of what studies get published are the people who complete the studies. That's right, Sanofi were the ones that chose which of their studies were published. If a company is given that much control, what do you think they would do? They would publish the studies that benefit them the most, the studies that favor the drugs they want to sell to up their profits. They wouldn't publish something that could potentially harm them and their profits.

The main point of the fact is that Big Pharma corrupts and controls the publication of this research so they can rush their medication to the market while going through as little testing as possible. This puts everyone's life in danger. They don't care about that though. All they care about is the profit.

Along with selective publication, another way the industry is controlled is through rigging the outcomes of these trials. Before 2000, these companies were not expected to declare what end points they measured while doing their trials. End point measurements are analytic measurement at the end of a chemical reaction. This is opposed to making the measurement during the reaction. What the companies would do during their trials is they would measure as many end points as possible and simply choose the one they thought looked the best. Once they did this, they declared the trial a success. If you measure all of your research this way, then you're bound to get a positive result at some point.

In the year 2000, the government made a move to stop this from happening. They made it a requirement for companies to register what they were measuring. Before the government did this in 2000, up to 57 percent of trials had a positive result. After 2000 when the companies were forced to declare what points they were measuring, only 8 percent of the trials showed positive results. If this evidence does not further cement the belief in the corruption of the medical industry, then what will?

## *Murdered by Medication*

It's hard to believe that something that is meant to heal us can actually end up doing more harm than good. A recent study claims that more than 250,000 people in the U.S. die every year from medical errors; however, other studies claim the numbers to be much higher, closer to 440,000 to be exact. The people in the medical industry are known to put their own needs ahead of the safety of their patients. There are many examples of this happening in the history of the medical world.

Opioid Crisis:

One of the most notable instances of this happening is with the opioid crisis. Opioids are addictive drugs that were pushed into the market, ignoring their addictive and dangerous properties, for the simple reason that they were extremely profitable. The sales of prescription opioids earned the medical industry up to

$11 billion in the U.S. annually. This nice profit helped Purdue Pharma, a big American pharmaceutical company, to overlook the fact that their drug was contributing to over 15,000 deaths by overdose.

Defective Vaccines:

Vaccines are something everybody knows about and not everybody agrees with. There are many rumors saying that they don't actually do anything to benefit us and there are also rumors saying that they can help us live better lives. The number of vaccines that are given to children has risen to extremely high levels. Children are vaccinated when they are born and we are given vaccines at intervals throughout our lives. A full lifetime's worth of vaccines can easily equal to 100. We allow this, and yet we do not trust them, and for good reason.

There are a lot of red flags surrounding the vaccines. One of the biggest is that any family in the U.S. is not legally allowed to sue any pharmaceutical company for an injury or death caused by the vaccines. These corporations cannot be legally held responsible for any harm caused by their vaccines. That is possibly one of the biggest red flags you can find.

In Australia, a child can be given up to 32 vaccines before they even reach the age of 1. Australians also have a vaccination schedule which requires them to get a vaccination at specific intervals in their life. In some places you don't have a choice on whether or not you want to be vaccinated.

Another thing strange about the vaccines is that a child is vaccinated at birth for hepatitis B. This disease is usually transmitted by sharing needles or having sex. Why are they vaccinating children for a disease that can only be transmitted through sex and sharing needles? Because it means profit. All of this adds up to a lot of profits for the Big Pharma.

The case of herd immunity is often made when discussing the importance or need of vaccines. The concept is that if the whole herd, in other words a very high proportion of the population, is immune to a certain disease, we can ensure that no one falls ill with disease and it will eventually die out. This is often used to justify the use of vaccinations. However, there are a few flaws in this concept.

In countries like the U.S. and Australia, a lot of people are flying in and out of the country on a regular basis. More often than not, a large part of the population includes tourists and yet none of them are checked for vaccinations. They could be bringing in any kind of disease which would go against the concept of herd immunity, but this concept is still used religiously by Big Pharma to justify their vaccinations. The concept of herd immunity is flawed and the vaccines are defective. The pharmaceutical companies know this and the government helps them get away with it by protecting them from legal actions.

Medical Errors:

It's not just drugs that kill people. Often, people are killed by the doctors or nurses themselves. These are medical errors. It's already been discussed that people make mistakes, but some errors cannot be excused. Many people have died in their hospital bed or during surgery because a medical professional made the smallest of mistakes. One such case was that of a little girl only 2 years old. She was diagnosed with an abdominal tumor. After various surgeries the tumor was removed and the little girl was declared cancer free. To be sure the doctors insisted that she go through her last trial of chemotherapy. Her parents eventually agreed.

It was a three-day treatment and on her final day the pharmacy technician prepared the intravenous bag. He somehow managed to fill it with 20 times the recommended amount of sodium chloride. The little girl was placed on life support a few hours after that and she was eventually declared brain dead. Three days later the parents had to say goodbye to their 2 year old daughter. She was fine. She had beaten cancer and was ready to live a full life, but one mistake ruined her chances at any kind of life.

This case is a sad one but it is not the only one out there. As mentioned above, 250,000 people die every year due to medical mistakes. Because of this, it is the third leading cause of death in the U.S. after cancer and heart disease.

## FDA Recalls

The FDA, Food and Drug Administration, is responsible for protecting and ensuring the public's health and safety. They ensure that drugs and food released to the public meet the health and safety standards. When anything that is released to the public is found to be dangerous to the people, it is recalled by the FDA.

According to the FDA, a drug recall is the best way to protect the people from a harmful or defective product. A recall is usually a voluntary action taken by the company who has the defective or harmful drug. They can take this action at any time to remove the entire harmful or defective product from the market. The thing that we should worry about is the fact that drugs with the potential to harm us are actually released to the public before being called back by the FDA.

A lot of drugs are recalled by the FDA and most of them we do not even hear about. Some of them are recalled for minor issues but these issues, no matter how minor they are, can cause serious harm to the public. These drugs are taken through a large amount of testing and yet they are still released with these defects.

## Pemoline:

This drug is also known as Cylert and it was on the market for a long time, from 1975 to 2010 to be exact. It was used to treat ADD and ADHD. The FDA released a warning that the drug can cause liver damage in 1999. The drug was later recalled completely.

## Bromfenac:

This drug was also known as Duract, and it was only on the market for a year, from 1997 to 1998. It was an effective pain killer. However, in the year it was on the market it caused 12 severe liver damage cases, 4 deaths, and 8 liver transplants. When it was released the drug was labeled with a warning that it should only be taken for 10 days. However, patients were being given a dosage for longer than 10 days. Those that died or suffered from liver disease were the ones taking it for longer than 10 days. The FDA was quick to recall the drug.

## Rofecoxib:

You will know this drug as Vioxx and it was on the market from 1999 to 2004. As you know, this drug increased the risk of heart attacks and strokes. It was responsible for up to 28,000 heart attacks in the U.S. It was reported that the drug caused 4 heart attacks per 1000 patients who took the drug. The company who manufactured the drug, Merck, recalled the drug voluntarily but not before it was given to more than 20 million people in the U.S.

## Sibutramine:

This drug was also known as Meridia and it was on the market from 1997 to 2010. It was an appetite suppressant, but it also caused heart disease and increased the risk of stroke in the people who took it. It was called another Vioxx before it was recalled by the FDA.

**Efalizumab:**

Also known as Raptiva, this drug was on the market from 2003 to 2009. It was used to treat psoriasis. It was recalled when they found out it caused progressive multifocal leukoencephalopathy. This is a rare disease and it is extremely fatal. It causes damage and inflammation in the white matter of the brain and the central nervous system.

There are many more drugs that have been recalled by the FDA. Some are just as dangerous as these and some not as much. Even though these drugs were eventually recalled and taken off the market, they still managed to get there in the first place. How can something so dangerous and fatal as these drugs get to the public? With all the tests and trials these drugs are taken through, they should be deemed unsafe before they even get the chance to see the light of day. The sad truth is that they are not. The big companies that manufacturer these drugs let them pass through the radar because it is not the health and safety of the public that they are thinking about. The only thing they are thinking about is the money they stand to make from potential sales of the drug.

The corrupt system is growing bigger and the risk for harmful drugs to reach the public only grows. We can't trust the people in the system because they are owned by it. If you ever think that your doctor or the pharmaceutical companies can be fully trusted with your life, just remember this: you being sick keeps them rich. Why would they cure you if that were true?

# Chapter 3:
# Fat and Weight Loss

The weight loss and dieting industry is almost as powerful and as profitable as the medical industry. There are always new dieting trends and weight-loss schemes coming out. There are always new reasons to spend your money on another way to lose weight. The weight loss industry has its own giant companies just like the medical industry. These companies have been around since the start of the weight loss and dieting trend. They've changed ownership and grown larger ever since then. One of these companies is Weight Watchers, which has rebranded and changed the name to WW.

Today the world is a competitive one and with every company out there coming out with a new and rewarding way to lose weight, can we really trust any of them? All of these options are so customizable and personalized, as the companies will have you believe. They will have you believe in the miracle diet that can make you lose weight while still enjoying what you're eating. If it sounds suspicious to you, then you're able to see through the façade.

Weight loss and the miracle diets are all a lie and all of these companies' goals are purely profit driven.

The weight loss market is probably one of the most profitable markets out there. In the U.S. alone profits grew from $69.8 billion to $72.7 billion annually. Their profits grew at a rate of 4.1 percent in 2018. The forecast says that their profits will continue to grow by 2.6 percent annually straight through to 2023. That's just the beginning. Prescription obesity drugs, which are used to suppress appetite and help with weight loss, earn up to $655 million per year. It's earned that much for a long time with its profits never falling or rising for that matter. Weight loss surgeries are growing at a huge rate in the U.S. In 2018, it's estimated that 239,000 bariatric surgeries were performed. This earned the market $5.98 billion. The growth rate for these surgeries is estimated to be at 5 percent per year.

The weight loss and dieting market goes up and down with profits and losses, however the profits are usually huge while the losses are small. Every company involved in this industry works hard to keep up with current trends. They try to lie to you and tell you that you need to eat a certain way in order to lose weight, but in most cases this simply isn't true.

# The Truth About Diets and Weight Loss

The weight loss industry would have you believe that weight loss can be gained by simply eating less and exercising more. This can be true in some cases, but not all of them. Many nutritionists believe that the answer lies in simply eating better and living healthier. There is no one perfect solution for everybody who wants to lose weight and be healthier. Everybody is different and we react differently to certain diets and exercise. That is something that most people in the weight loss industry won't tell you, because they'll lose money that way.

Here are some things that these companies won't tell you that could potentially help you live a healthier lifestyle and lose weight on your own.

**1: Skip the Diet**

It sounds weird at first, but diets can actually harm you more than they can help you. Most of the time people won't stay on a diet for their whole life. They'll diet until they've lost the weight they want to, then they'll stop or they'll try different diets until they can find one that works for them. This can cause a lot of problems. This kind of lifestyle leads to something called weight cycling in which someone will diet until they lose weight, drop the diet, then gain all of the weight back again. They'll start the process over and over. Diet and lose weight, drop the diet and gain weight, then go back on the diet again. Doing this long term can lead to some health issues such as chronic inflammation, high cholesterol, and blood pressure levels.

The best way to avoid this is to avoid diets. It's much more sustainable to develop a healthier lifestyle than it is to live on a diet. Work exercise and strenuous activities you enjoy into your life. Create a meal plan with healthier foods that you actually like and live off of that. Don't go on a diet for a few months to drop a little weight only to gain it again. Most diets are not sustainable, therefore the weight loss is not sustainable. What is sustainable is a healthy lifestyle.

**2: Food Diaries Can Help**

A food diary can help you keep track of your meals and can even help you lose weight more efficiently. What you eat is a big part of losing weight. It's very easy to eat the wrong thing. The point of the food diary is to document everything you eat throughout the day. In a couple of weeks you could see an unhealthy pattern forming and change it before it does any damage. If you notice that you always eat a snack in between breakfast and lunch, that might mean that your breakfast isn't filling enough and you need to change it. Perhaps you notice that you aren't eating any fruits or that all of your vegetables are in one meal a day and not spread out. A food diary can help you notice these things and change your habits.

You can keep a food diary the old way with an actually book and pen, or you can download an app on your phone. Any way that suits your lifestyle. Make sure to be honest with yourself and write down everything you eat or it won't work.

## 3: Portion Sizes Are Everything

It doesn't always matter what you're eating; it's the amount of it that matters. Giving up food doesn't help if the portion of food you're eating is too big. Even if you give up unhealthy food like soda and candy, the healthy food can still make you gain weight if you are overeating. The portion size of your food matters a lot more than what type of food you're eating.

Depending on your height, weight, and age, you burn a certain amount of calories a day even without exercising. You burn these calories by doing nothing. If you eat more calories than your body is burning and you're not exercising, then you will gain weight. If you eat fewer calories than your body is burning and you're exercising, you will lose weight. You can eat more calories than your body is burning and use exercise to get rid of the excess and more if you want. Just remember that portion size is important. Don't just watch what you eat, keep an eye on how much you eat.

## 4: Exercise!

As mentioned in all of the previous steps, exercise is the key ingredient to a healthy and sustainable lifestyle. Being more mindful of what and how much you eat, but it doesn't really matter if you aren't keeping active. The more active our body is, the more calories we burn, and the healthier we are. An active daily routine can lead to disease prevention and help you live a longer life.

There are many different ways you can keep yourself active. You can join a gym or yoga program. This is something that can keep you motivated because there are other people there to encourage you. Another way is to take up an active hobby that you can enjoy and work into your daily life. This can be anything from biking, to ice-skating, or even dancing. There are plenty of activities that can easily be added to your daily lifestyle that help keep you healthy and active. Give them all a try and see what works best for you. Remember, even the most effective diet is useless without exercise.

## 5: Allow Yourself a Cheat Meal

Although we all want to eat and live healthy, it's hard at first. It's hard to give up on all of those tasty meals we used to have. We know that this food isn't good for us, but that doesn't stop it from being delicious. It's important not to be too hard on yourself. You like eating pizza, a glass of that sugary drink is really refreshing, and nothing beats a bag of chips. There is no kidding ourselves about this.

We have to cut this kind of food out of our daily life because we know it is not good for our health. That doesn't mean you have to cut it out of your life completely. Allow yourself a chance to indulge. Have a cheat meal at least once a week. Allowing yourself to eat something unhealthy once in a while can actually help you on that weight loss journey. When we completely starve ourselves of the few things that we like, we are setting ourselves up for failure.

Allow yourself one meal a week in which you are allowed to cheat. Eat whatever you want. Have a pizza, or a burger, or even just some chips. Make sure it is only one meal. Some people give themselves an entire day to cheat. This can harm your end results, but one meal won't set you back. Treat this as a reward for being so healthy the rest of the week. As long as you don't go overboard, then you should be alright.

## 6: Resist the Empty Plate Urge

We all have the same urge to eat everything on our plate and leave it empty. We don't actually have to do this. If you choose not to eat everything on your plate, you could be starting a healthy habit that can help you in your efforts. This strategy could end up saving you up to 100 calories per meal. It doesn't sound like much in the grand scheme of things, but if you do it every day, then it will start to add up. It's a small gesture but it will have a big impact. All you have to do is resist the urge to eat that last piece of fruit or that last bit of meat.

## 8: Eat More Vegetables

Vegetables are good for you, we all know this. They are filled with fiber, they're low in calories, they're a good source of water, and they can make you feel full faster. A good habit for meals is to make sure that at least half of your plate consists of veggies. Make sure you eat the veggies first because they'll fill you up and save you from eating a lot of calories. This strategy can also help you cut down on the rest of the food which may not be unhealthy but is probably not as healthy as the vegetables.

## 9: Brush After Your Meal

This is another small gesture that can have a big impact. Brushing your teeth after you've finished eating can get the taste of food out of your mouth and signal to your body that you are done eating. This way you can cut down on late night snacks. We all sneak a snack every now and again. You won't want to do that after you've cleaned your teeth. Get into the habit of cleaning your teeth the moment you've finished eating and you will see the results.

## 10: Self-care

Most importantly, you have to put yourself before everything else. The diet may not be working for you and it may be harming your health, so drop it. You don't have to be obsessed with losing weight especially if it's hurting you along the way. You don't need a diet to lose weight, you just need to care for yourself. Ignore the scale for now and work on getting your life together so you're more active and eating healthier. Once you've got it all working out for you, then you can check how the numbers on the scale are.

It would be easy if there was just a diet that actually worked for everyone. That's what those big companies would have you believe. However, it's not true. Everybody is different. One diet might work for one person but that doesn't mean it will work for you as well. Diets are a lie fed to us by the weight loss and diet industry. Diets don't work when it comes to a healthy life and weight loss. Having healthy habits and living an active lifestyle is the only way to lose weight and keep it off. We may have to change our lives in order to make them healthier and sustainable but in the end, we are rewarded more for it.

## Lies About Weight Loss

We've all been told a thing or two about weight loss and dieting. These things are 'facts' or things we have to do if we want to lose weight. We're led to believe that if we don't follow these certain steps, then we won't lose weight no matter what. All of these things are lies. I'm going to list these ridiculous so called 'facts' so you know to avoid listening to the people who tell you to do this.

### 1: Fewer Calories

Some people will say that the fewer calories you consume, the better. This is not only untrue but it can also set you up for failure. The less we eat during one meal, the more likely we are to overeat during the next meal. Not only that, but we can actually cause ourselves harm because we aren't giving our bodies enough energy. Yes, it is good to eat less but if you eat too little, you are basically starving your body of the energy and nutrients it needs to get through the day. Restricting the amount of calories you eat is not good. It's better to eat healthier and less food while still giving your body what it needs instead of starving yourself for quick results.

**2: Six Meals a Day**

This is on the opposite side of the scale. Instead of eating fewer calories, people spread their daily calories into six small meals a day. This can be a good idea for some people, but for others it can be bad. The reason is that everyone has a different version of what a small meal is. If your six small meals a day turn into six not so small meals a day, you'll end up overeating. Also, a Canadian study has found that this method of splitting your daily calories into six meals doesn't have that much of an effect. The research said that if you eat six meals a day rather than the usual three, it can actually make you want to eat more. If you want to try out this method then I suggest you learn everything you need to know about it first so you can follow it properly.

**3: No Carb! No Fat!**

A healthy lifestyle is all about balance. You can't have balance if you're taking things away from your diet. It's simple, if you take one thing away you could end up eating too much of something else. Some dieting trends ask you to eliminate an entire food group like low-fat or low-carb diets. These are the worst diets. If you cut fat out of your diet you could end up eating more carbohydrates. Carbohydrates are known for stimulating insulin which is a fat storing hormone. However, if you cut carbs out of your diet you could end up feeling sluggish or become constipated.

The trick is to monitor how much of each food group you eat, but you cannot remove an entire food group altogether.

## 4: Skip the Meal and Have the Juice

This is a bad idea. Some advice might tell you to swap out your meals for a juice instead. This juice is supposedly healthy and better for you. However, that juice is most likely filled with sugar and it won't fill you up. You're just going to be hungry later and end up eating more calories than you should be. It's actually better that you chew your meals because, believe it or not, chewing is a form of exercise and can actually get your metabolism going. Chew your food, don't drink it.

## 5: A Tablespoon of Coconut Oil a Day

I'm sure you've heard it once or twice. If you eat a tablespoon of coconut oil a day it can help you lose weight. Some people think this is a miracle cure for weight loss, but it's not. Coconut oil is saturated fat. It's basically like lard. Do you really want to eat a tablespoon of lard every day? One tablespoon of coconut oil equals 12 grams of saturated fat and 117 calories. The American Heart Association suggests that we limit our daily intake of saturated fat to 13 grams a day. One tablespoon of coconut oil is basically the entire recommended limit of saturated fat a day. If you have more you are putting yourself at risk of a heart attack.

Skip the tablespoon a day and just use it in your cooking. You'll probably end up eating a lot less of it.

## 6: Eat this Every Day

Some diets will tell you that you must eat a certain food every day or even with every meal. These diets should be avoided at all costs. A diet that puts focus on a certain food can be dull and lacking in certain vitamins. A diet may tell you to have a grapefruit with every meal. For the first few days it might be okay, but you'll get bored of the taste after a while and it will stimulate your cravings for some other food. If your cravings are stimulated then there's more of a chance that you will cheat on your diet and it will all be for nothing.

## 7: Exercise and Diet Apps

Ignore these and keep them off of your phone. Some apps claim they can calculate how much you can eat based on how many calories you burned during exercise. Just because an app tells you that you can binge eat doesn't mean you should. It's actually impossible for an app to be able to tell how many calories you burn while exercising. People exercise at different strengths and speeds which means they burn calories at different rates. One app on your phone cannot tell you how many calories you have burned, which means it can't judge what you can eat without gaining weight. Just stick to your own diet and exercise and trust that you're eating right.

## 8: Have a Big Breakfast

One of the most commonly heard dieting facts is that you have to eat a big breakfast. It's true that breakfast is the most important meal of the day. It gives us the energy we need for most of the day and fuels all of our early morning activities. However, a big breakfast is not necessary for this. It is possible to have too much fuel in the morning.

Instead of eating a huge breakfast in the morning, choose a normal sized breakfast with a good amount of protein in it. Protein is the food we need to energize ourselves. Things like eggs or Greek yogurt can give us all the energy we need for the day without the possibility of overeating.

## 9: Supplements

There is some information out there that would have you believe you can burn fat just by taking vitamin and mineral supplements. This is false, of course. You may need these supplements to replace the vitamins and minerals you aren't getting in your diet, but they do not act as miracle weight loss drugs. If you need to take them, then by all means do so but don't think they'll magically burn fat and solve your problems.

**10: Detox for Weight Loss**

There are a lot of detox teas or juices out there that all of these weight loss and diet companies try to sell us. They'll tell you all sorts of things like detoxing can help you lose weight. There is no scientific evidence out there that supports this information. Our bodies naturally cleanse themselves every day. What really matters is what we put into our body. Just eat natural and let your body to its job. There's no need to waste your money on those 'natural' detox products when your body already does the job.

There it is. These are the common lies a big weight loss and diet company will try to tell you so you spend more money on them. In the grand scheme of things, the weight loss industry is no different than the Pharmaceutical industry. They don't care about you. They care about profit. You're just another client who they can try and fool into spending money on countless diets that won't work. The need for a diet is probably one of the biggest lies they can tell. Diets aren't sustainable. A healthy, active lifestyle is sustainable and more affordable. Don't become a slave to the dieting industry and the scale.

The true information is out there for you to see. It is the same situation with your doctor. You don't trust him completely with your health, so you shouldn't trust these weight loss companies with your health either. Take it into your own hands.

# Chapter 4:
# Foods Your Body Needs and the Pyramid of Lies

The very first food pyramid was created in 1988 and it was seen as an important guideline to eating and living healthy. These dietary guidelines were written in great haste and virtually no trials nor tests were run to support them. When the first food pyramid was created there was no scientific evidence to support it. The public was spoon fed the belief that the food pyramid is the best guideline to live by. They stated that if you only ate what and how the pyramid told you to, then you would live a healthy life. However, given the fact that there was no evidence to support their claims, we can safely assume that the pyramid of food was a lie.

The pyramid of food is a visual guide used to show people what food is bad for them and what food is good for them. It takes the shape of a pyramid with the good food groups being at the base and the bad food groups occupying the top. The first food pyramid encouraged people to consume more carbohydrates and to avoid fat. These guidelines were, of course, successful. It decreased America's consumption of fat by 15 percent. This sounds like a huge success. However, with the consumption of fat reduced, why did the obesity and diabetes rates increase? The food pyramid and these dietary guidelines were meant to increase the overall health of the population. If that's the case, why is it continuing on a downward spiral with more and more Americans becoming obese and diabetic? The answer is simple; because the food pyramid is part of the big industries that rule the world.

Big Pharma, the weight loss and dietary industry, and the food industry are all part of one big machine. The food pyramid is just part of their lies to control how much the public spends and how much profit they make. Evidence for this is there for those who are looking for it.

Every five years the Dietary Guidelines must be reviewed by a panel of experts as required by the legislation. The panel must consist of 15 different experts in obesity, cardiovascular disease, nutrition, pediatrics, and public health. This panel of experts, however, cannot be trusted, and neither can their review of the Dietary Guidelines. This is because the process of selecting the panel of experts is heavily influenced by lobbying. Yes, the same lobbying we see in the medical industry happens here as well. This is evidence that the dietary system cannot be trusted. Big companies like the American Meat Institute, the Wheat Foods Council, the Soft Drink Association, and the Salt Institute are the companies behind the lobbying. These and other companies work hard and spend big to ensure that the Dietary Guidelines appear in their favor. The only reason they would invest money into something like this is if they can stand to gain more money from it. With the right influence, these companies can control what the public deems healthy. Through that, they can control what the public chooses to buy. All valid reasons to assume the Dietary Guidelines and the food pyramid are lies.

Up until recently, it was considered business and social suicide to even consider that the Dietary Guidelines may not be trustworthy. Researching it or suggesting an alternative to the system was considered crazy. Now there are some people who are willing to break down the lies and expose the Dietary Guidelines for what they are. One important contributor to this new movement is Walter Willett. He is the chairman of the Department of Nutrition at the Harvard School of Public

Health. Walter Willett is the spokesperson of a long-running diet and health study. These studies are extremely comprehensive. The studies have cost more than $100 million and have included 300,000 individual civilians. According to Walter Willet, all of the data from these studies contradicts the current "low-fat is good for your health" beliefs.

There are good fats and there are also bad fats, but the current food pyramid would have you believe that all fats are bad. They have been focused on making sure the public cuts fat out of their diet. However, most scientific evidence available to us has proven that has only caused more problems for the public's health. Walter Willett believes the lie that all fat is bad for you has contributed to America's rising rates of obesity.

The people who are willing to perform studies like this are helping the public to combat the rule these big companies have over us. It's sometimes hard to believe just how deep the corruption goes. All of these companies are run by politics and profits. They don't care about the public. We're all just customers with money. One fact that can show how shady the business world is involves the Heart Association. The Heart Association is a non-profit organization in the United States. They fund cardiovascular medical research and they try to educate the public on proper cardio care in order to reduce the risk of cardiovascular disease and stroke. The Heart Association was also founded by a company that makes and sells alternatives to butter. Those sets of circumstances are suspicious. They warn the people of the risk that the fat in butter poses for your heart and then they make money selling you alternatives to butter. This is another reason why no product or information that comes out of these big companies can be trusted.

The main point is that the food pyramid and the Dietary Guidelines have done far more bad than they have good.

America has the highest obesity rate in the world and the diabetes rate has only gotten worse. There were about 30 million diabetics in the year 1985, and now it's predicted that there is going to be 438 million diabetics in 2030 and a lot more pre-diabetics. This is all because of the misguided food pyramid.

# What You Should Be Eating

We've spoken about a low-carb diet earlier. Although you shouldn't completely eliminate a food group from your diet, you can minimize your consumption of certain foods. The low-carb diet is by no means a new discovery. It's been around for over a century, but it has recently gained some traction. The low-carb diet is a good choice for combating obesity and diabetes. There are foods that diabetics shouldn't consume under any circumstances and then there are foods that are okay for diabetics to eat. Some of these foods go against the guidelines set by the food pyramid.

Butter, cheese, fish, all meat, olive oil, and all organs are foods that diabetics can eat freely. Bread, oats, flour, rice, sugar, starches, and juice are all foods that should be removed from a diabetic's diet. The foods that should be removed from a diabetic's diet actually form the base of the food pyramid. That means these are the foods you can eat freely according to the Dietary Guidelines. Vice versa, the foods that a diabetic can eat freely are restricted according to the food pyramid.

There's no problem with having fat in your diet. There are healthy fats that are actually good for you. The best way to add fat into your diet is after you've lowered your carb intake. So increase your healthy fat intake after lowering your carb intake. It's that simple. The current American diet consists of high fat and high carb which is the main cause of the obesity and diabetes epidemic. If you increase your fat but keep eating the same amount of carbs, you'll also end up on the standard American diet. So this step is probably the most important one.

It sounds weird when you hear that you should actually be eating more fat. It's not just any fat you're eating. There are good fats which provide good nutrients for your body as well as bad fats that harm your body when you consume too much of it. However, the same thing can be said of carbohydrates. There are good and bad carbohydrates but the problem is that too much of both can be harmful. The reason you shouldn't remove fat from your diet is because when you do you're removing nutrients your body needs and most of the time you're replacing the fat with something far more harmful.

When fat is removed from a food, something replaces it. Sometimes whatever is used to replace the fat is worse than the fat itself. Take cream cheese, for example. Low-fat cream cheese consists of 15 percent carbs, while regular cream cheese only has 4 percent carbs in it. Reading the label on certain foods might increase the time it takes you to shop, but you can see for yourself exactly what you're buying that way.

The fear of fat is the cause of the Dietary Guidelines we've been blindly following for nearly two generations. However, these guidelines have no scientific evidence to back them. For these two generations we've been told that reducing our fat intake, especially saturated fats, will decrease our risk of cardiovascular disease and reduce our cholesterol. Yes, saturated fat does reduce the cholesterol in our bodies but it mainly reduces the good cholesterol. Yes you heard that right. There is such a thing as good cholesterol and we need it in our bodies.

Reducing your consumption of saturated fats reduces HDL in your body which is the good cholesterol. Reducing saturated fats also makes LDL which is the bad cholesterol. Low-density lipoprotein, or LDL, is the majority of cholesterol we have circling in our bloodstream. Scientists proposed that there was a link between the LDL and heart disease. This link is the reason the Dietary Guidelines have insisted on the public lowering their fat intake. However, further studies have shown that you can reduce the amount of LDL in your body by reducing your fat intake, but this did not decrease the number of heart disease cases or mortality rates.

In short; LDL, which is bad, carries cholesterol from the liver to the body and the organs. HDL, which is good, carries the cholesterol from the body back to the liver for disposal. There have been some new studies done on reducing the LDL by having a high-fat diet and a low-fat diet. In these studies the high-fat diet was better at reducing the incidence of heart disease.

My advice would be to not ignore the food pyramid entirely, as some of its information is correct. However, not all of it can be trusted. Take all of its advice with a grain of salt. Make sure you do your homework and find out what's best for you to eat rather than trust that someone else cares enough to give you the right information. The best diet by far is the low-carb and high-fat diet.

Here are some simple tips and habits that can change the way you eat and better your lifestyle:

- When you think you're hungry take a moment to ask yourself, "Am I really hungry or am I just bored?" Learn the difference between hunger and boredom. This can lead to a lot of snacking.
- Try eating a wide variety of foods. If your meals get dull or plain, then you might end up overeating something more enjoyable. Your meals can get boring if you eat the same things all the time. Make sure your meals are healthy but try to experiment with new tastes.

- Fill your plate with non-starchy vegetables. The right vegetables are filled with fiber and they can help you lose weight and stay active. Make sure at least half of your plate is filled with non-starchy vegetables. Eat as many vegetables as possible to make sure it doesn't get bland or dull.

- Introduce a wide range of low-sugar fruits to your diet. These can make great midday snacks if you find you are feeling a little hungry in between meals.

- Make bigger dinners at night so you can save some for lunch the next day. If you make twice the amount of food you can have a good healthy dinner and then a good healthy lunch the next day. This saves time and it saves you having to decide what to have the next day. Obviously you shouldn't do this every night, as your meals could end up getting boring.

- Remember to eat healthy fats such as olive oil, butter, and avocados.

# Chapter 5:
# The Cardio Myth: Exercise Smart

There are a lot of myths and lies surrounding exercise. Everyone always has the 'right way' to exercise. The magazines, TV shows, and YouTube videos, are all lying. Everybody wants to be the one that knows what you can do to lose weight, but most of the knowledge out there is just a myth.

It's time that you knew the truth. There are some big lies out there, but the thing is that they seem legit enough that we automatically believe them. The logic is there, but it's still wrong. Just because it sounds right doesn't mean you should believe it. I'm going to shed some light on the biggest exercise myths so you know what to believe and what you shouldn't believe.

## The Big Lies

### 1: Cardio Burns Fat

This is probably one of the biggest lies. You've probably heard it before. Cardio exercise is the best exercise for burning fat. It sounds like it makes a lot of sense. It gets your heart going, it makes you sweat, and it burns a lot of calories. However, it's not the best exercise for burning fat or losing weight. The thing with cardiovascular training, things like jogging, skipping, cycling, or running, is that your body can quickly adapt to it. This kind of training seems hard at first but it only takes a short while before your body adapts to the exercise. This means that you'll be burning fewer calories every time you exercise. In order to keep up and keep burning fat at a high rate, you have to increase the intensity of your cardio training more and more every time you exercise. This can be dangerous and is less effective over time.

Another bad thing about cardio training is that as soon as you stop, so does the fat burning. You're only burning calories during the exercise. Other forms of training, such as weight training, still burns calories long after you've stopped exercising. To sum it up, cardiovascular training is a good form of exercise and it's a great way to stay active, but it is by no means the best exercise for burning fat. There are a lot more effective ways to burn calories and fat than cardio.

**2: Walking Isn't Exercise**

Of course walking is exercise! Any time your body moves you are exercising. Walking was the only form of exercise our ancestors got. Before we all were on diet trends and gym memberships we were walking. It's a great form of exercise. It falls into the cardio category but it's still exercise. Some people out there will have you believe that walking isn't proper exercise and that you need to jog and run everywhere, but they're wrong. We should all walk every day. A walk a day can keep the doctor away. Seriously though, walking is good for mental health, cardiovascular health, calorie burning, fat loss, overall well-being, and it is a sustainable activity. That's more than you can say for a lot of forms of exercise.

**3: You Have to Exercise Every Day**

No you don't. Whoever said that is obviously lying. This statement also depends on what you consider to be exercise. As I said earlier, any time when your body is moving and being active can be considered exercise. With that logic, we're already exercising every day. It is good to stay active. You can be active every day and exercise every day, but that could take the form of many things like walking your dog.

You don't have to go to the gym or do a full exercise routine every day. It's actually better for weight loss if you allow your body some rest time. What happens when you exercise is you're actually tearing and stretching your muscles. That's why you feel strain while you exercise and that's why you're sore the next day. This is good. What this allows your body to do is repair itself. While your body is repairing itself, it's burning more calories and fat. However, in order for your body to repair itself you have to give it the chance. That means resting for a day or so.

By all means, be active every day. Take the stairs instead of the elevator, be bubbly and move around a lot. Even if you're standing in line at the grocery store or in front of the stove in the kitchen, you can be more active. Dance a little, sway your body from side to side. Anything that gets your body moving gets your metabolism going and helps you lose weight. You don't have to go to the gym every day to exercise every day. Your body needs that rest in order to repair itself. Once it's repaired, you can go back to your normal exercise routine, but remember not to put too much of a gap in between your workouts. There is such a thing as too much rest.

## 4: More Pain, More Gain

This information is not only wrong, it is also dangerous. It's very easy for someone to be misled by this saying. You should never work out until you hurt yourself. There is a difference between straining yourself and hurting yourself. If you exhaust your body or train too hard you could end up seriously hurting yourself. You need to know your limits and stay under them. You will gain without pain.

That being said, you also need to know that feeling a little strained doesn't mean you should stop because you're in pain. It's important to know the difference. You will feel strain while exercising, but you can't stop the moment you feel the strain.

This part can be difficult, but once you find your limit you'll know when you have to stop and when you can keep going.

## 5: If It's Fun, Then It's Not Working

Who thought up this? It sounds like it makes sense, right? Exercise is sweaty and it's hard work. It shouldn't be fun. If it's fun for you then you aren't doing it right.

That's completely wrong. Exercising doesn't have to be a chore. You don't have to dread the moment you need to exercise. There are forms of exercise that you can find enjoyable and it's actually better if you enjoy it when you exercise.

Certain activities and hobbies are enjoyable and they do fall into the category of exercise. Things like biking and rollerblading are exercise and they could be enjoyable activities. The more you enjoy exercising, the more likely you'll keep at it for years. The lie everyone keeps telling about how exercise needs to be strenuous and you can't enjoy it is probably one of the most harmful lies out there.

You can enjoy your exercise and it's actually better if you do. So have as much fun with it as you can!

## 6: Weight Training isn't for Women

Some people would have you believe that women shouldn't do weight training. This is a silly lie. Why shouldn't women do weights? Some people might believe that weight training is meant for men, but we can argue that women can gain more from weight training than men. Weight training can help women increase their bone density, help with their mental well-being, fat loss, and body composition. One of the best advantages women can gain from weight training is the offsetting of osteoporosis.

An understandable fear that most women have with weight training is that they'll gain muscle. Not all women actually want to bulk up like men, but you don't have to worry because this won't happen easily. Women don't have the level of testosterone that men do, so they simply won't be able to gain muscle that easily. At least, not like men do, anyway. There are a lot of good things women can gain from weight training, so silly rumors like this shouldn't stop them from doing it.

### 7: You Have to Work Out in a Gym

I don't know who thought up this lie, but I hope it sounds as stupid to you as it does to me. Of course you don't have to work out in a gym if you want to get fit or lose weight. Our ancestors never had a gym to work out in and they did fine on their own. Nature has a gym of its own. The world around you can be your gym if you know how to use it. There are hiking, biking, and running trails, and each one can work out your body in different ways. There are also plenty of sports and hobbies out there that don't require a gym membership, things like swimming and rock climbing. So, to answer, no you don't need to work out at a gym if you want to lose weight or get fit.

### 8: Yoga isn't an Actual Workout

Yoga can be a pretty relaxing activity. It's supposed to be great for your mental and emotional health, but there are plenty of other benefits beyond relaxing and chilling out. Yoga is strenuous if you haven't done it before. It's a great workout with many benefits. Yoga has been known to correct posture imbalance and strengthen skeletal tissue. It can also encourage better breathing habits as well as act as an offset to injury. Yoga has even been connected to improving blood flow and heart health. Yoga is indeed great for relaxing but it's also a very beneficial workout.

### 9: Weight Training Can Help You Get Big

It's actually a lot more complicated than that if you want to gain muscles. Weight training does help, but there's more to it than that. You have to build your whole lifestyle around it if you want to gain some proper muscles. It takes a lot of effort. You need to eat the right food, plan the right workout, and be dedicated if you actually want to bulk up in the right way. It takes far more than just lifting weights a few times a week or when you have time. It's a whole lifestyle.

**10: Lose Weight First, Then Exercise**

This is probably one of the biggest and worse lies out there. It's kind of a silly one as well. Why would anyone think that you have to lose weight before you can start exercising? The main reason anyone would exercise is because they want to lose weight. Sometimes this lie is told to people who are well above the weight they should be or people who are obese. They're told that they can't start exercising until they've lost a bit of weight first. Then they're put on a diet to lose that weight but as mentioned before, diets don't work and they especially don't work if you're not exercising as well.

You don't need to lose weight before you can start exercising. Yes, you won't be able to do anything extreme until you've lost a little weight, but there are a lot of exercises out there suitable even for people who have never exercised before. As mentioned above, any time your body is active you are exercising. Don't listen to those people who say you need to diet and lose weight before you can exercise. Just start exercising. Do it today, right now. Don't let anyone stop you. The sooner you start, the sooner you can reach your goals.

*The Biggest Lies*

The lies above, although harmful to the world of exercising and fitness, are only small white lies. There are far more harmful myths out there. These big lies can make someone's life harder if they're trying to lose weight or get fit. They can even discourage someone and stop them from reaching their goals. Now we're going to expose these lies for what they are.

**1: Calories are Calories**

Calories are all anyone ever talks about when it comes to eating healthy. One of the most harmful beliefs is that all calories are the same, so you don't have to worry about what calories you eat, only how many of them you eat. Everyone is sold on the idea that they can eat what they want as long as they stay under their set calorie limit. This limit is predetermined based on their age, weight, and height. People have been made to believe that they just need to stay under the limit and then they can eat what they want. This is an extremely harmful myth.

The truth is that not all calories are the same. Some calories are more harmful than others. It's the same as having good fats and bad fats. There are good calories and bad calories, and yes it matters which ones we eat. The calories we consume give our bodies different hormonal effects. For instance, the calories you get from an M&M will give you a different hormonal effect than the calories you get from an avocado. These hormonal effects are why simply counting calories is not good enough for any kind of end result.

Your body needs fat, protein, and carbohydrates to remain in hormonal balance. There are good and bad versions of all these food groups, and you need to find a proper balance between all of them. Each one of them has a different effect on your body. Fat slows down your digestion and it increases your satiety. Carbohydrates make your blood sugar rise. Protein helps your body store body fat which is used to provide energy. We need each of these food groups for our bodies to run the way they're supposed to.

When we eat carbohydrates, our blood sugar is raised but this provides us with energy to use. The energy provided by these carbohydrates is usually used immediately, with sugar being used first. However, if you eat too much of this food group then the remaining sugar in your body that can't be used for energy is stored as body fat. This storage is controlled by the hormone insulin.

When we eat protein, all of that body fat which was stored by the insulin is then used for energy. This is done by the hormone glucagon. This hormone acts as a counter to insulin so that we don't end up with too much stored body fat. Without protein, our bodies wouldn't be able to mobilize the stored body fat into energy.

Eating fat basically helps us to feel full. It slows down our digestion and increases our satiety. Fat also slows down the rise of your blood sugar which in turn slows down the release of insulin. Eating fat can help you to limit the amount of fat that your body stores while making your body think it is full so you stop eating.

As you can see, all of these food groups help your body stay healthy and balanced. All of the things these food groups accomplish have nothing to do with the amount of calories you eat and everything to do with balancing the hormones in your body. This should be more than enough evidence to prove to you that overeating calories is not the cause of fat gain or an unhealthy lifestyle. The only cause is not giving your body the right balance of the three food groups it needs.

## 2: The Scale Determines Your Health

This isn't exactly a complete lie or myth, but it's not a whole truth either. People believe that the weight you see on the scale determines how healthy you are overall. While this is true with some extreme cases such as obesity, it simply isn't fully true with everyone else.

We end up spending half our time looking at the scale and feeling discouraged and unhappy with the result we see. We eat healthy and work out every day but the number on the scale doesn't always change. Sometimes the scale won't show you results even when they are there. When we exercise to get fit or lose weight, it doesn't always show on the scale straight away. The best way to avoid unnecessary disappointment is to ignore the numbers on the scale and focus on your body's composition. Your body composition is the measure of how much of your body is muscle tissue, how much of it is fat, and how much of it is water. Then there's even how much of it is bone.

What we need to do is look at our body composition. Instead of working on lowering the number on the scale, we need to work on lowering the proportion of stored fat in your body to muscle. It often happens, especially with women, when they've followed their diet precisely and they work out every day but then they step on the scale and find that they haven't lost any weight or that they've even gained weight. This can be discouraging if you don't know what's really happening. You see, muscle weighs more than fat. When you're cutting away at the fat in your body, then that fat is usually replaced with muscle. Seeing the number on the scale go up or stay where it is can lead you to believe that what you're doing isn't working and you're making no progress when that simply isn't true.

It's better to focus on how you look in the mirror rather than what the number on the scale is. You'll decrease in clothing size, but the scale may stay the same. Ignore the scale and focus on your body's composition if you want to see true results.

## 3: A Comfortable Workout Works

There is no such thing as a comfortable work-out. You can't stay in your comfort zone and expect to give your body what it needs to lose weight and get fit. There is a whole industry of fitness and health built around this one myth. There is no way you can achieve results without pushing yourself beyond your comfort zone.

This lie takes many forms. You can casually walk every day and lose weight. You can have abs in eight minutes. Do this 3 minute workout once a day and you'll lose weight. All you need to lose weight are shake weights. All of these and more are lies. If you want to achieve proper results it is far more difficult than that.

Every single time you put your body through a workout, it will learn and adapt to it. This means that the next time you do the same workout your body will react differently and even do it easier. This will yield few to no results over time. Once your body adapts to a certain workout, the only way to counter it is to intensify your next workout.

Every time you go for a run, you have to run faster and further. Every time you lift weights you have to increase the weight or the number of times you lift them. Whenever you do any kind of exercise, the next time you have to increase the intensity in some way. This is the only way you can counter your body's ability to adapt.

When we exercise we are asking our body to adapt to what we're doing. Basically, if you run 5 miles a day in 20 minutes, then that is what you're asking your body to adapt to. You're asking your body to change itself so you can consistently run 5 miles a day in 20 minutes. Your body's fat and muscle and your fitness level will change to match this goal only. It will never change if you don't change the intensity. Your body will reach this adaption after some repetition but once it does, there will be no further change or gain.

Therefore, a comfortable workout will never help you reach your goals. You have to push yourself. Every time your body adapts to a certain workout, you have to intensify it somehow. Don't worry though, you only have to do this until you reach your goal. Once your body has managed to adapt to the fat and muscle percentage that you want, then all you need to do is maintain that level. You won't have to intensify your workout anymore but you can't allow yourself to relax too much either. In order to maintain your body's adaptation you have to push it to the point you've reached every time you work out. If you allow yourself to get lazy or slack off, then you will only see yourself moving backwards.

Now that you know all of the lies the world of exercise and fitness have been spreading, you can keep your sights on the few truths there are. There are a few things you can do to improve your health and lifestyle. You don't need to listen to the lies people tell you even if they appear to be an expert in their field. Remember that they have something to gain from you believing what they tell you even if what they're telling you is a lie.

The only truths you need to know are these few I have told you. If anyone tries to tell you otherwise, then be very wary of them. Most often you'll find that they just have something to sell to you.

# Chapter 6:
# The Cholesterol Myth

We've touched on cholesterol earlier in this book. I'd like to talk about it a little more. There is a big myth surrounding the word and it can be very harmful if you don't know the full truth behind it. Cholesterol has become a bad word lately. It's understandable considering the connections it has to heart disease, strokes, and heart attacks. There is a definite connection between the two, that part is not the myth, but there is so much more to the story that isn't being told. What I told you earlier will appear again here, but I will be expanding on the science of it and the exact differences between good cholesterol and bad cholesterol. I'll also explain properly why we need cholesterol in our bodies so we can work past this myth once and for all.

In order for us to live healthy and happy lives, our bodies need to be in perfect balance. We can't eliminate cholesterol from our bodies entirely and expect to be in balance. The truth is that we need cholesterol, and more harm than good will come from eliminating it completely. The cholesterol levels in our bodies are usually used as an indication of our heart's health. However, the relationship between our cholesterol levels and the health of our heart is not set in stone. Some people who have a high cholesterol level don't seem to be affected by it at all, while others have been affected directly by their cholesterol level. This can be explained only by the fact that there are two types of cholesterol.

There are two different types of lipoproteins that our body uses to carry cholesterol from one cell to the other. One form of cholesterol is called low-density lipoprotein, or LDL, and the second form is high-density lipoprotein. The amount of both types you have in your body can be measured with a blood test, and obviously it matters how much of each one you have.

### *The Bad Cholesterol - LDL*

Low-density lipoproteins are considered to be the bad cholesterol. The LDL cholesterol directly contributes to the buildup of fat in the arteries which is known as atherosclerosis. Having this condition causes the arteries to be narrowed. There is a direct connection between the narrowing of your arteries and the increased risk of strokes, heart attacks, heart disease, and peripheral artery disease, also known as PAD.

Having too much of this cholesterol in our bodies can be extremely harmful. Our best way to control how much of the bad cholesterol we have in our bodies is by controlling how much of the good cholesterol we have.

### *The Good Cholesterol – HDL*

High-density lipoproteins can be considered the good cholesterol. Where with LDL we should have less of it in our bodies, with HDL we can argue that it's better that we have more of it.

Higher levels of HDL could help our bodies lower the levels of LDL. Experts in the subject have found evidence that HDL carries the LDL cholesterol from the arteries and back to the liver. Once it is there, the liver breaks down the LDL until it is passed from the body. However, HDL does not rid the body of all of the LDL cholesterol. HDL only carries about one-third to one-fourth of the LDL cholesterol in our blood to the liver. It cannot carry the remainder. There is evidence to suggest that having a higher HDL level can help protect us against things like heart attacks and strokes. Studies have also been done that show people with low levels of HDL are at a greater risk of heart disease.

### *Triglycerides*

Having high levels of LDL or low levels of HDL cannot contribute to heart disease all by itself. Another thing that plays an important role are triglycerides. This is the most common type of fat we have in our body. What this fat does is it stores excess energy it gets from your diet. This fat is also linked to the risk of heart disease.

When you have a high level of triglycerides in your body combined with either a high level of LDL or a low level of HDL, you are at more risk of having a fatty buildup in your arteries. This is a direct link between this and heart attacks or strokes.

# What You Need to Know About Cholesterol

Cholesterol is a waxy substance in your body that we all get from two sources. We get it from our liver, and from the food we eat. Cholesterol travels through our bodies in the bloodstream. It usually travels in fatty bundles known as lipoproteins.

We have low-density lipoproteins or LDL, which is the bad cholesterol. This kind of cholesterol can slow your blood flow, clog your arteries, and create blood clots. When your LDL levels are high, you are at a greater risk of heart attacks, strokes, and heart disease.

We also have high-density lipoproteins or HDL in our bodies, which is the good cholesterol. This type of cholesterol removes the bad cholesterol from your blood and takes it to your liver where it can be broken down and removed from the body. When your HDL levels are high you are at a lower risk of heart attacks, strokes, and heart disease.

That is the basic information that you need to know about cholesterol. Cholesterol is solely tied to the cause of heart disease, so it is targeted by doctors and medical professions. Although having the wrong levels of cholesterol in your body can raise your risk of heart disease, it isn't the only thing that can cause it. There are many other things that can increase the risk of heart disease in anyone. People tend to single out cholesterol as the main cause because it can be treated with drugs, diet, and exercise. However, most of the other things that can cause heart disease can also be easily controlled and countered.

## *Other Causes of Heart Disease*

### 1: Smoking

This one is a no brainer, really. Smoke from cigarettes can give the body a lot of problems. One of those problems is raising the cholesterol. Not only does smoking raise your cholesterol levels, it also forces your heart to work harder. All of this puts you at risk of heart disease.

### 2: Obesity

It's not just obesity in general that can raise your risk of heart disease. To be more specific, it is the size of your waist that can raise your risk of heart disease. This is true even for people who have no previous risk of it.

### 3: Blood Pressure

It shouldn't come as a surprise that the higher your blood pressure is, the higher your risk of heart disease. When you have high blood pressure it can make your heart muscles stiff. There are a lot of things in life that can raise your blood pressure, but all of them can be controlled and eliminated as needed.

## 4: Diabetes

Diabetes is a problem all by itself and even if you're controlling your blood sugar levels, just the fact that you have diabetes raises your risk of heart disease.

## 5: Being Inactive

We need to be physically active in order to lower the risk of heart disease. Whether it's because of your job or your lifestyle, not everyone can be as physically active as they should be. When we exercise, we lower our blood pressure and help strengthen our hearts. So if we aren't getting enough exercise, then we weaken our hearts and raise our blood pressure which in turn raises our risk of heart disease.

## 6: Triglycerides

We've already discussed how this type of fat in our bodies is directly connected to heart disease. It's linked with cholesterol and this type of fat in your blood comes from the food you eat. Too much of it can cause a buildup in your arteries. We can control this by controlling how much of it we eat. Lowering the levels of this fat in our bodies will lower the risk of heart disease.

As you can see, there are far more causes of heart disease than just the cholesterol in our bodies. However, the big cholesterol myth will have you believe that the main and only cause of things like heart attacks and strokes is the level of cholesterol in your body. Nobody wants to tell you about the different types of cholesterol and why you need one type of it rather than just getting rid of all of it. It's easier for people to tell you to just cut down on the fat and lower your cholesterol levels, but it's far more complicated than that.

While all of the main causes of heart disease are somewhat controllable, there are some other causes that simply can't be controlled.

### 1: Age

There's no denying that the older you get, the more at risk you are of heart disease. Yes, there are things you can do to lower the risk as you get older. A good diet and active lifestyle lowers the risk at any age. However, as you get older, the risk will get higher and there's not much control over that.

### 2: Family History

We can't escape or control our history. Unfortunately, if your parents or grandparents had heart disease, then the chances that you'll have it as well are much higher. That's something that can't be controlled.

### 3: Gender

Yes, gender plays an uncontrollable factor in the risk of heart disease. If you're male you have a higher chance of having a heart attack at a young age. However, if you're female your risk of heart disease rises after menopause. Both men and women are at risk of heart disease, however men are at a greater risk at a young age than women are.

## Controlling Your Cholesterol Levels

Here's what we know so far: among other things, having a high level of LDL cholesterol in your body or a low level of HDL cholesterol can put you at risk of heart disease. What we also know is that the levels of good and bad cholesterol in your body are directly connected to your diet. What we eat determines how high or low our cholesterol levels go. It's safe to assume that by controlling what we eat, we can lower our LDL levels and raise our HDL levels as we see fit.

You don't need your doctor to prescribe you any kind of drug. You don't need help from any of those money grabbing health and weight loss companies. All you need is to know what you're putting in your body and learn how to control your cholesterol levels.

## *Foods that Lower LDL Levels and Raise HDL Levels*

One of the best ways to lower your LDL levels is to eliminate foods in your diet that have it. However, you can also add foods that counter the cholesterol and carry it out of the body in different ways. Some foods you can eat contain polyunsaturated fats; these are responsible for directly lowering LDL levels. Other foods combat it in a different way. Some have soluble fiber, which binds the LDL cholesterol in your digestive system so it is passed from the body before it even has the chance to enter the bloodstream. There are these and other ways that the food in your diet can help lower the LDL in your body.

### 1: Vegetable Oil

You can use oils like sunflower, canola, and other forms in place of things like lard or butter. These vegetables oils directly lower your LDL levels.

### 2: Oats

Oats or oat based foods contain a valuable ingredient, soluble fiber. Probably one of the easiest ways to lower your LDL levels is to have a bowl of oats or oat based cereal in the morning. It will give you 1 to 2 grams of soluble fiber a day.

### 3: Nuts

There are a lot of studies that show the benefits of nuts when it comes to your heart's health. All of these studies say that nuts are good for your heart, specifically peanuts, almonds, walnuts, and some others. If you eat at least 2 ounces of nuts a day, it can slightly lower your LDL levels.

## 4: Eggplants and Okras

These vegetables are a must have in any diet. They are low in calories and they contain soluble fiber which helps to directly lower LDL levels.

## 5: Strawberries, Citrus Fruits, Grapes, and Apples

These particular fruits are rich in pectin. Pectin is a type of soluble fiber which directly lowers your LDL levels. For your five fruits a day, make sure they're these fruits.

## 6: Whole Grains

Whole grains, like barley, are similar to oats. They can lower LDL levels in your body because they contain soluble fiber.

## 7: Fish

Adding fish to your diet, especially fatty fish, can help lower your LDL levels in multiple ways. One way is by replacing other meats with fish. Meat has saturated fats which boost LDL levels. If you eat fish a few times a week, you'd be replacing the LDL boosting meat and it will be giving you omega-3 which lowers LDL. Omega-3 does this by lowering the levels of triglycerides in your bloodstream.

## 8: Beans

Beans are useful for lowering LDL levels and for people who are trying to lose weight. Beans are rich in soluble fiber so they directly lower LDL. Beans also make you feel full faster so they are a must have in any weight loss diet.

## 9: High-fiber Fruits

Fruits that are high in fiber not only lower your LDL levels but they can also raise your HDL levels. Add fruits like pears and prunes to your diet in any way you want.

## 10: Avocados

This fruit isn't new on the scene of food, but it has gained recent popularity. It's high in fiber which naturally helps keep cholesterol levels in check and it contains a certain type of fat known as monounsaturated fat. This is a healthy fat and it can directly lower your LDL levels.

## 11: Red Wine

Yes you read that correctly. Red wine, when drunk in moderate amounts, can slightly raise your HDL levels. One glass of red wine a day for women and two glasses a day for men have been shown to lower the risk of heart disease among other benefits. This is a tricky one, though. You shouldn't just start drinking a glass a day straight away. The effectiveness of red wine is dependent on the other factors of your lifestyle. If you have high levels of triglycerides, then drinking red wine could actually do more harm than good. If this is the case, other drinks such as grape juice or just grapes can contain the same effects as red wine.

## 12: Soy Products

Soy products are mostly on the market for vegetarians but that doesn't mean that others can't eat them, too. If you add soy products to your diet, you can reduce the amount of meat you consume. We already know that meat can raise our cholesterol levels, so this is a good step to counter that. Although the fact that your HDL levels rise and your LDL levels lower is probably not directly connected to soy products, but rather as a result of eating soy instead of meat.

## 13: Chia and Flax Seeds

Flax seeds contain omega-3 and fatty acids. It's a favorite for vegetarians and helps to lower LDL levels in the body. Chia seeds are also a good source of omega-3 and are great for fiber. It directly lowers LDL levels and your blood pressure.

It's better to consume flax seeds once they are ground. If you eat them when they are whole, they won't be digested properly and your body won't absorb any of their nutrients. Chia seeds tend to gain a slimy texture once they are wet. If you don't want this, then rather consume them directly or add them to your baking.

# Chapter 7: Stop Counting Calories

Life is all about balance. Having a good and healthy lifestyle requires the perfect balance. For perfect balance we must understand what our bodies need and what we don't need. We must also understand that there is no good in eliminated something from our lives but we should rather try and see the good and bad of everything. There's no need to eliminate something completely when there is an option to only keep the good while removing the bad.

We've discussed the good and the bad in almost everything. Just like there are good and bad cholesterol, there are also good and bad calories. This, however, is not a widely known fact and that has harmed many people in many different ways.

## The Calorie Myth

The current wide-spread method of weight loss is simple and easy to follow. All you have to do to burn fat and reach your goal weight is to eat less and exercise more. It sounds so easy that it's almost unbelievable. Well, that's because it doesn't work. This is an outdated and under studied method that has managed to squirm its way into society and for some reason hasn't been kicked out yet.

One of the most common low calorie diets is the 1200 calories a day diet. A lot of people are on this. They count calories religiously and exercise until they're sore every day. They do all this and yet for some people they don't see any results. In fact, many people work themselves to death eating less and exercising more just to lose weight but instead find themselves somehow gaining weight. This is because it isn't as simple as eating fewer calories, because not every calorie is the same. Most people dedicate their lives to managing their weight but if you don't actually know what the right thing to do is, then at the end of the day nothing you do will matter and that's the cold, hard truth.

The calorie myth states that all calories are equal and simply reducing your consumption of all of them will help you lose weight. By this logic, that means that if a glass of soda and a glass of freshly squeezed orange juice had the same amount of calories then it won't matter which glass you drink. Both glasses will have the same effect on you because they have the same amount of calories. This logic doesn't just sound ridiculous, it is ridiculous. It doesn't take an expert to realize that a glass of orange juice is far healthier than a glass of soda even if they contain the same amount of calories. This is the simple difference between good and bad calories.

The problem we find in diets, such as the 1200 calories a day diet, is that people on the diet are allowed to eat whatever they want as long as they stay in the allowed number of calories. Basically, someone could drink a glass of soda instead of orange juice because they'll still stay within their calorie limit. A person could stay under 1200 calories a day but it doesn't matter if all of the calories they're consuming are bad calories. The counting calories method is one bound for failure and there's no denying that.

There are of course other factors besides the fact that calories can be both good and bad. As mentioned before, the body needs to be perfectly balanced. It needs certain nutrients in order to function properly.

One of the main things in our bodies that assists us with weight loss is our metabolism. With a slow metabolism we're more likely to gain weight, and with a fast metabolism we're more likely to lose weight. In order to have a fast metabolism we need energy and we get that from food. If we starve ourselves of this food then we slow down our metabolism and ultimately gain more weight because of it. This is still connected to the difference between good and bad calories, of course. Certain foods can cause our metabolism to slow while other foods can speed it up.

In short, it doesn't matter that much how many calories we eat. What matters most is the type of calories we eat. We need to focus more on what we eat rather than on how much we eat. This is how your body works: when you eat more calories your body will automatically burn more calories, and when you eat fewer calories your body will automatically burn fewer calories. That's the simple science of it. It happens that way to everyone every time they go on a low calorie diet.

The 'calories in and calories out' system does still work to some extent. You can still end up overeating the good calories. Setting for yourself a calorie limit isn't exactly necessary, especially one so constrained as 1200 calories a day. However, you do need to set yourself some limits so you don't end up overeating.

### *The Importance of Quality over Quantity*

Your body is like a system. It's like a machine and it has certain needs if you want it to keep running at an optimal rate. It's like a machine that runs on oil. The machine needs a certain amount of oil to run, and if it gets less oil than it needs it won't run properly. Your body needs a certain amount of calories in order to run properly. If it doesn't receive the correct amount, then it will slow down and eventually break down.

The problem with the modern world is that people don't change what they eat when they go on a low calorie diet. They simply eat less of it. They're still eating the same bad food but they make themselves feel better about it because they aren't eating a lot of it. That's what most people do and it is the first step on the path to disaster.

By eating less food we eventually end up starving our body of the food it needs to run properly. Once we do that we become hungry, tired to the point of lethargy, and we can even become depressed. This is a downward spiral. We can't keep this up forever. No one can essentially starve themselves forever. When we eventually crash we will not only stop eating less, we might even end up eating more than we were before we even started the diet. When this happens, and it will happen, you will end up not only gaining weight but you will gain more weight than you had before. This is the quantity over quality diet.

If your body requires a certain amount of calories to run properly, then it only makes sense that we feed our body that exact amount of calories. No more and no less. This way our bodies can run the way they're supposed to and give us the energy we need. It's not just about giving our bodies the correct amount of calories it needs. It's mostly about the kind of calories we give it.

There is evidence that by feeding our bodies the good calories, we help it heal itself. When we feed our body the correct calories it heals our brain, starts creating the correct hormones, and sets our gut back on the right track. When we heal our system we will start consuming and absorbing the right amount of calories and we will also start burning more of those calories. This all relies heavily on the type of food you give your body rather than the amount.

Protein is one of the best calories you can give your body for two beneficial reasons. The first reason is that protein fills you up better than other food groups. You'll end up eating about 100 calories of protein and you'll already feel full but if you eat

100 calories of carbohydrates, you'll still be hungry. The second and most beneficial reason you should eat protein is that it stops your body from burning muscle tissue instead of stored fat. When we reach the right amount of calories for our body to consume, our bodies will end up burning all of it. A big portion of the calories that our bodies burn comes from stored fat. If there isn't any stored fat for your body to burn it will start burning muscle tissue. This is very bad and you don't want this to happen. Adding protein to your diet can stop this from happening.

Protein is just one form of the good calories you can feed your body. You need to focus on the good food and how you can feed your body more of it. This is the quality over quantity diet.

Overall, it does matter how many calories you put into your body. However, the amount of calories doesn't matter nearly as much as the type of calories does. We can't starve our bodies of what they need. We need to at least give our bodies the exact number of calories it requires to run properly, no more and no less. Once we are only giving our body the calories it needs, it will end up burning up all of them and then some. This is why it is required that we are giving our body the good calories and not the bad. Then we can use smart exercise to fill in the rest of the gaps and speed up weight loss. The most important thing to remember out of all of this is if you want to lose weight, starving your body isn't the answer. Giving your body exactly what it needs is the right way to go about it.

## *Exercise Smart*

Along with the calorie counting myth, we get the exercising more myth. People often say that you should eat less and workout more. They encourage you to work out every day and push yourself beyond your limits. While there is some truth in this, there is also a potential to hurt your body badly.

The main exercise options are aerobic exercises that are suitable for burning calories. These exercises include things like jogging daily. This is a good way to go about things, but there are better ways. Exercising smart involves low-impact but high-intensity exercises for about 20 minutes, up to once or twice a week. You can do more by exercising harder.

Most of the exercise advice that people have these days focuses primarily on burning calories. Burning calories isn't enough, though. Your body is already burning calories itself. The best exercises we can do involve trying to improve upon the calorie burning system we already have. The best and easiest way to do this is by building up our metabolism and adjusting our hormonal balance. We can do this through exercise as well as food.

We can achieve this by engaging all four of our muscle fibers during exercise. We have four types of muscle fibers. During an exercise such as jogging, we are only engaging one type of muscle fiber. In order to engage all four types of muscle fiber, we must produce more force for our bodies. This means that we need to exercise harder, move faster, and just have more intensity in our exercise routines. When we do this we won't have a need to exercise every day because you'll get quite a few days worth of exercise in just one day.

The reason we want to engage all four muscle fibers is because it will force our body to produce certain hormones. Our bodies will be forced to produce adrenaline, growth hormone, epinephrine, and noradrenaline. All of these hormones are clog-clearing hormones and they work to free up the energy that is being stored as body fat.

Your body naturally tries to use as little energy as possible when performing any given task. The muscle fiber's job is to conserve energy at all costs. If you lift something heavy, your body will use as little muscle fibers as possible to do so but if it sees that you require more muscle fibers, then it will give you more. It does this until eventually you end up using all four of your muscle fibers. You have to push your body past its comfort zone if you hope to use all of your muscle fibers. However, you don't want to do this the wrong way or you'll end up using too much energy which means you won't be able to exercise as much. That's where knowing how to exercise the smart way comes in handy.

Things like taking the stairs, going for a daily walk, or even a bike ride are all fine for general health and keeping active. These types of exercises generally work on your duration and frequency but they don't work on your resistance. The best chance you have of losing weight is to build up your resistance. You can accomplish this with targeted resistance training.

What you want to do is some high-intensity interval training for about 10 minutes, two times a week. That's all you need to do. Eccentric muscle workouts are the best because they leave your muscles feeling sore for a few days. You take those few days to rest, then once the sore feeling is gone you can exercise again. This will leave you about two days a week to exercise and if you're doing it right, that should be enough.

An eccentric workout is when your muscle is worked while it is lengthened. It's basically the opposite of lifting weights because all of eccentric workouts involve lowering weights. An eccentric movement is like when you're lowering your body into a squat or if you're lowering a dumbbell after you've lifted it. Studies show that during eccentric movement every muscle fiber in your body is at its strongest.

When you're exercising, make sure to do a full body workout. Get every single part of your body involved. People usually have leg days, arm days, and chest days. That works for some people, but to get the best results you have to get your whole body into it in one day. So work out your chest, legs, arms, back, shoulders, and abdominals all in one for the best possible workout.

## *Eating Smart*

We've abolished the calorie myth. We've shown you that calories are not the same and that what you eat matters far more than how much you eat. Now we can talk about what you should be eating. It's all very well me telling you that you shouldn't eat bad calories, but how are you supposed to know what the good calories are? I won't leave you to guess. I can tell you what qualities a food must have if it falls into the category of good calories.

## 1: Nutrition

This is a given ingredient in any healthy food, or good calories. If a food can provide you with the nutrients you need, then it should be added to your diet. You want nutrients such as vitamins, essential amino acids, minerals, phytonutrients, and essential fatty acids. The more nutrients there are per calorie, the better.

Sweets, starchy foods, and sugary drinks usually have few nutrients if any and carry a lot of calories. Low-sugar fruits, nuts, protein, non-starchy vegetables, and seeds usually contain a lot of nutrients and fewer calories.

## 2: Satiety

If a food is able to make you feel fuller faster, then that is good for any diet. A food that makes us feel full has satisfied our appetite. There are many foods out there that don't satisfy our appetites and keep us eating more. Things like pizza do this. We will end up consuming a lot of calories without feeling full and this is a bad thing for anyone trying to lose weight.

Foods like broccoli, protein-rich meat, and tuna can make us feel full while not eating too many calories.

### 3: Non-aggressive

There are calories out there that trigger the production of glucose in our bodies. With the increased production of glucose, our body is more likely to store anything we're eating as body-fat. We call these aggressive foods. It's best to avoid the foods that do this and stick to the non-aggressive foods.

### 4: Digestibility

The harder it is for your body to digest a food, the better. If the body cannot efficiently digest a certain food, then it's less likely that food will be converted into stored body-fat. Our bodies can't digest fiber so it can't be stored as body-fat. Protein is also difficult for the body to digest; therefore it is passed through the body instead of being stored as body-fat. The body does try to digest these foods but after spending calories, so with little luck it eventually gives up on the food and it is passed. These foods are better to eat because they will cut down on the amount of body fat that is stored inside you.

Starches and sugars are usually easy to digest, so they are always stored as body fat. Fats are easily converted but they also have other desirable factors that make them a good addition to any diet, in moderation of course.

# Chapter 8:
# Eating to Prevent Cancer

When it comes to the risk of cancer, there are very few causing factors that we can control. Things like genetics are completely uncontrollable. If there is a history of cancer in your family, then you are at a greater risk of getting cancer yourself and there isn't much you can do about it unfortunately. However, some studies suggest that up to 70 percent of your risk of cancer throughout your life is within your control.

Avoiding known cancer causing products is fully within our control. Things like smoking cigarettes, drinking alcohol, exercising regularly, and keeping your body at a healthy weight are all under your control and making the right choices can lower your risk of cancer. Having the right diet can also lower your risk of cancer. We all know that there are foods out there that are known as cancer causing foods. There are also foods you can eat that can help you lower your risk of cancer.

What you eat or don't eat is a big part of your health, even to the point where it could lower your risk of cancer. Even if you have a history of cancer in your family, making small changes to your lifestyle can still lower your risk.

## *Red Meat and Processed Meat*

For a few generations now red meat, such as pork, beef, and processed meats such as bacon and ham, have been labeled as cancer causing foods. This information has shaped the dietary guidelines and the pyramid of food since the beginning. The World Health Organization has classified red meat and processed meat as a Group 1 carcinogen. This basically means that it is known to cause cancer in people who consume certain amounts of it each day. Of course, this has not stopped the public from consuming these products. According to research, the average American diet consists of 4 and a half servings of red meat a week. Even more, about 10 percent of the population consumes two servings of red meat a day.

The science behind this information used to seem pretty solid. We were told that research showed that there were certain chemicals in processed and red meat that made the food carcinogenic. These chemicals were both natural and added during processing. According to this research, a chemical in red meat and processed meat known as haem is broken down in the gut once the food is consumed. When we break down this chemical, it forms other chemicals known as N-nitroso. The research showed that the N-nitroso chemical damages cells that line the bowel. This ultimately leads to bowel cancer. This research also suggested that the chemical was more present in processed meat than red meat and so processed meat should be avoided at all times. However, recent information has put doubt into this research. Recently, an international collaboration of researchers, through various trials and studies, found that this information which has shaped the American Dietary Guidelines for generations stands on shaky evidence.

The research involved looking through trials that linked red meat to cancer. The researchers also looked at articles that examined the links between red meat and incidence of cancer and mortality. Every study found that there were little to no links between red meat and disease or death. The quality of evidence that has been used to form the Dietary Guidelines was very low.

I should say that even though the links between red meat, processed meat, and cancer are low, they do still exist.

However, most of the research that has been done proving that red meat and processed meat cause cancer was done on large groups. In the region of science, evidence gained from large group studies is weak evidence. If a link was found in a few people amongst a large group, then how can they suggest that a single person will benefit from cutting out these products?

The evidence on both sides of this argument can be considered weak. However, even with knowing the risk of cancer that comes with eating these products, it hasn't stopped anyone. Red and processed meats are still a large part of the average American diet. Even if these products aren't the big cancer causers as we've been told all this time, it still wouldn't hurt to cut down on them.

## Cancer Causing Foods

Red and processed meats have 'clogged up' the pool of cancer causing foods. Most of the talk about cancer causing foods has basically surrounded these two products, but there are several more that can share the same blame. Avoiding these foods and drinks altogether or limiting your consumption of them will reduce your risk of cancer.

There are so many articles and research papers out there telling you that they know what foods cause cancer. Everyone seems to have the facts. With there being so many facts out there, how are we supposed to determine which facts are true and which ones are false? We do it by looking at what we know. For a food to be labeled under cancer causing, it needs to be carcinogenic and for that to happen there has to be strong evidence that consumption of a food or drink can lead to an increased risk of cancer.

### 1: Alcohol

This is a given choice. There has been plenty of research and a lot of evidence to prove that alcohol causes cancer. To be specific, the more alcohol you drink, the greater your risk is of contracting head, liver, breast, neck, colorectal, and esophageal cancer.

When we drink alcohol it produces a chemical compound known as acetaldehyde. This chemical compound may cause damage to your DNA and this is what leads to the risk of cancer.

Although it's better to avoid alcohol altogether, experts have come up with an allowable daily limit. That is one serving of alcohol a day for women and two for men. Serving sizes vary depending on the type of alcohol. A serving of wine would be 5 oz., beer is 12 oz., and liquor is 1.5 oz.

**2: Diet food and drinks**

Diet foods and drinks have gained popularity at an alarming rate. They're supposed to be a better and healthier way for us to enjoy some of our favorite guilty pleasures. Recent studies have shown that certain diet foods and drinks may not be as healthy we are lead to believe.

Diet foods and drinks are made with the use of artificial sweeteners. This eliminates the use of the harmful refined sugar but adds something even more harmful. The European Food Safety Authority has done up to 20 separate studies that found one of the most commonly used artificial sweeteners, aspartame, as the cause of a range of illnesses including cancer. There are various other sweeteners that have been linked to the cause of cancer, such as saccharin and sucralose.

Diet foods and drinks are dangerous and they don't really do that much for our health. It's best to avoid them completely.

**3: Refined Sugars**

While you're avoiding diet foods and drinks, it's also best to avoid refined sugar products as well. There are multiple reasons to avoid refined sugar. One of the main reasons is that it tends to spike your insulin levels, which in turn feeds cancer cells. Fructose-rich products such as high fructose corn syrup or HFCS is probably the most harmful. Studies have shown that cancer cells can easily and quickly metabolize HFCS in order to spread. Sodas, cereals, cookies, pies, cakes, juices, sauces, and other processed products have a lot of HFCS in them along with other forms of refined sugar. These are popular products that are filled with cancer causing ingredients.

## 4: GMOs

GMOs or genetically-modified organisms and the chemicals that are used to grow them have been proven to contribute to the rapid growth of tumors. GMOs are in basically everything. The only way to properly avoid them is to stick with certified organic, locally grown food, and non-GMO verified foods. Try to buy foods that are produced naturally.

## 5: Microwave Popcorn

Placing a bag in the microwave for a few minutes for a nice snack may seem convenient, but it is also more harmful than you would think. The bags of microwave popcorn are lined with chemicals such as perfluorooctanoic or PFOA. This chemical has been linked to the cause of testicular, liver, and pancreatic cancer. There are several independent studies proving the chemical causes tumors. There is another chemical in popcorn known as diacetyl that is linked to lung damage and eventually lung cancer.

## 6: 'Dirty' Fruit

Dirty fruit is basically any food that is verified and certified organic and pesticide-free. You may think that you're being healthy by buying that bag of apples or grapes, but for all you know they are covered in pesticides which are cancer causing chemicals. Conventional produce is a no go. Studies have found that up to 98 percent of conventional produce are covered with these cancer causing pesticides. It's best to make sure your fruits are organic and verified pesticide-free.

## 7: Refined White Flour

Refined flour is commonly used in a lot of processed foods. The worrying thing about this ingredient is the excess amount of refined carbohydrates in it. A recent study that was published in the Cancer Epidemiology journal showed that refined carbohydrates, like those found in refined flour, are linked to an increase in the risk of breast cancer. This was a significant increase of 220 percent. Foods that are high-glycemic have been proven to raise blood sugar levels. Something like this directly feeds cancer cells and helps them grow and spread.

## 8: Soda Pops

Soda pops are generally unhealthy, as they are loaded with many forms of refined sugar. They're also filled with food chemicals and colorings. Soda pops directly feed cancer cells and they acidify the body. The most common chemicals used in soda pops such as caramel color and 4-methylimidazole are also directly linked to causing cancer.

## 9: Hydrogenated Oil

Hydrogenated oil is mostly used in processed foods as a preservative. The use of hydrogenated oil allows companies to extend the shelf life of their processed products. However, this ingredient has been linked to altering the structure and flexibility of cell membranes. This can raise the risk of many diseases including cancer.

Recently, a few companies have made steps to fade out the use of hydrogenated oil, but trans fats are still used in processed food and it isn't that much better.

## 10: Farmed Salmon

Farmed salmon is a high risk cancer food as it is loaded with chemicals in order to lengthen its shelf life. It lacks vitamin D which is something you should get from fish such as salmon. It's also often contaminated with pesticides, flame retardants, antibiotics, and polychlorinated biphenyls or PCB. All of these chemicals are carcinogenic. Avoid farmed fish at all cost and buy fresh, because fish is a really good addition to any diet as long as it isn't contaminated with chemicals.

## 11: Sugar

Sugar is loosely implicated as a cause of certain kinds of cancers. Otto Warburg, a German biochemist, found that cancer cells often used sugar to fuel their growth. This study was done in the early 20$^{th}$ century. The Warburg effect, which was established after his discovery, suggests that if you starve the body of sugar and things that can be converted into sugar like carbohydrates, then you could in turn starve the cancer cells. This is how the ketogenic diet was created. This diet reduces the amount of carbohydrates you consume to about 10 percent. It also increases your fat consumption by 70 percent. This supposedly works to slow down and starve the cancer cells. However, the effectiveness of this diet has not been scientifically proven to help slow down cancer cells and it comes with a lot of other health problems if not done properly.

The association between the increased risk of cancer and sugar is still there. It could help to cut down your consumption of sugar. When most people do this they tend to replace sugar with artificial sweeteners which have the same effect as sugar. Both of them should be avoided or taken in moderation if at all possible.

## 12: Very Hot Drinks

It sounds strange, but it's true. The evidence for it is sparse but it is there. Studies have been done that show drinking hot beverages, such as tea and coffee, can raise your risk of esophageal cancer. However, you don't have to cut these beverages out of your diet. You just need to wait for them to cool down first. If your beverage is hotter than 140 degrees Fahrenheit, or 60 degrees Celsius, then it is putting you at risk of cancer. Any temperature lower than that should be perfectly fine.

The reasons for a hot beverage to increase our chances of getting cancer are unclear. The evidence is there, but the exact cause is still unknown. It's believed that the raised risk in cancer may be linked to the damaged caused by the heat blanching our throat's cells.

Don't let this information put you off drinking any hot beverages. In fact, certain types of tea are good for your health and can even help you lower your risk of cancer. All you have to do to safely enjoy these beverages is wait for them to cool down before drinking them.

## 13: Burnt or Charred Food

Meat or food that is cooked at too high a temperature, burnt, or charred can raise your risk of cancer. If you burn your toast, you could be raising your risk of contracting cancer. If you like your meat well-done or barbecued, then you could also be increasing your risk. When meats are cooked at high temperatures or cooked to the point where they are burnt or charred, they start to form chemicals that may change your DNA when you eat it. This can lead to a higher chance of getting cancer.

If you are used to eating a large amount of meat that is fried, well-done, barbequed, or even slightly charred, then you are raising your risk of pancreatic, prostate, and colorectal cancer.

You can avoid this by slow cooking your meat at a low temperature. You could also bake, boil, or braise your meat instead. Some evidence has shown that marinating your meat before you cook it could help lower your risks.

Making these small changes to your diet can lower your chances of contracting any kind of cancer significantly. Some foods should be removed from your diet altogether, while other foods should be eaten in moderation. The key to any well balanced diet is moderation.

# Cancer Preventing Foods

Just like there are foods that can increase your risk of cancer, there are also foods that could lower your risk. You can eat your way to health and to a low risk of a variety of cancers. For example, a traditional Mediterranean diet could help lower your risk for many different kinds of cancer. This diet is rich in vegetables, fruits, olive oil, and healthy fats. These foods are on the list of foods that lower your risk. Even if you have a history of cancer in your family, you can still lower your risk by changing your lifestyle for the better.

Of course, there are other factors involved in the prevention of cancer, such as lifestyle, body weight, and how active you are. However, you can change your risk by a small amount just by changing your diet. You should still try to change your whole lifestyle for the better, as it will increase your chances of cancer prevention by a much more significant amount.

### 1: Fruits and Vegetables

It's recommended that we all eat at least five different fruits and vegetables a day. I think I speak for everyone when I say that not all of us manage to reach this limit. However, adding a variety of farm fresh, natural fruits and vegetables to our diet can help better our health in many different ways, including lowering the risk of cancer. I am, of course, talking about what we call whole foods. For example, a whole, unpeeled apple is far healthier than apple juice.

These are certified natural, fresh, and verified pesticide and preservative free. All of those chemicals are used to preserve the food's shelf life but, as we've already discussed, they also raise our chances of contracting cancer.

Once you've managed to find fruits and vegetables that fall under the whole food category, then you can add them to every aspect of your diet.

Add fresh cut fruit to your cereal in the morning. You can add cut fruit to your oatmeal, or Greek yogurt for a nice healthy start to the day. For lunch you can have fruit as a side or even some raw vegetables. A salad packed with vegetables with a side of fruit is extremely healthy. If you have snacks during the day, then make it a fruit or raw vegetables. And for dinner, you can fill your plate with fresh or frozen vegetables. Make sure at least half of your plate is made up of veggies.

**2: Healthy Fats**

It's been proven that having a diet high in fat can raise your risk of contracting cancer. However, just like almost everything else, there are good fats and bad fats. While the bad fats can raise your risk of cancer and leave you unhealthy in many other ways, the healthy fats can help to lower your risk of cancer.

Trans fat should be avoided at all costs and saturated fats should be limited as much as possible. Unsaturated fats should be added to your diet and used in moderation. Unsaturated fats are the healthy fats and you can find them in olive oil, avocados, nuts, and fish. Omega-3 is a fatty acid and it is one of the healthiest unsaturated fats you can add to your diet. You can find an abundance of it in tuna, salmon, and flaxseeds.

## 3: Antioxidants

A diet high in antioxidants can help lower your risk of various cancers. It's mostly plant based foods where you'll find an abundance of nutrients known as antioxidants. These help to boost your immune system which protects from many diseases, including cancer.

You'll mostly find antioxidants in fruits and non-starchy vegetables, but there are other foods that carry them too. Keep your eye out for foods with this nutrient and add them to your diet.

## 4: Fiber

Fiber is a key ingredient to keeping your digestive system properly clean and healthy. A diet that contains fiber can help keep cancer causing compounds from moving through your digestive tract and stop them from doing any harm. Fiber can be found in several food groups but it's mostly found in fruits, vegetables, and whole grain foods.

## 5: Green Tea

Green tea is a tasty beverage and it's good for many different health problems. Green tea is especially useful as part of an anti-cancer diet. The reason is because it's a powerful antioxidant. Research has found a chemical called epigallocatechin-3 gallate in green tea. This is a non-toxic chemical that acts directly against an enzyme called urokinase which is a crucial ingredient for cancer cells to grow.

Green tea is a known cancer fighting food and it can help you fight against breast, lung, liver, pancreatic, skin, and esophageal cancer. Add a cup of green tea to your daily routine because just one cup contains 100 to 200 milligrams of this cancer fighting chemical.

## 6: Garlic and Onions

Garlic and onions are not world-wide favorite foods. In fact, they're more of an acquired taste and if they are used, they're used sparingly. However, you should consider using them as abundantly as possible. Research has shown that onions and garlic are able to block the formation of nitrosamines. Nitrosamines are powerful carcinogens that are able to target multiple parts of the body.

The chemically active sulfur compounds in garlic and onions can help you fight against colon, breast, and liver cancer. So don't just add them to your diet, add as much of them as possible. The more you add, the stronger your defense against the cancer cells.

## 7: Tomatoes

Lycopene, a type of antioxidant, is a powerful cancer fighting food and tomatoes contain a lot of it. Research has shown that this type of antioxidant is even more powerful than vitamin E, beta-carotene, and alpha-carotene which are all cancer fighting foods. Eating tomatoes can help protect against certain cancers such as lung cancer and prostate cancer. Make sure to cook the tomatoes before you eat them, as this helps release the Lycopene and makes it easy for your body to access.

## 8: Olive Oil

Olive oil is a monounsaturated fat, which is a healthy fat, and it is widely used in Mediterranean countries for cooking and as a salad dressing. Recent research has shown that the risk for breast cancer in Mediterranean countries is 50 percent lower than in other countries where olive oil is not as widely used. The evidence that makes this a cancer fighting food isn't as strong as with other foods, but it's worth adding it to your diet anyway.

**9: Cinnamon**

Cinnamon is well known across the world for its many health benefits. One of those health benefits includes blocking the spread of cancer cells. There have been several tube-tests and animal studies that show how cinnamon and cinnamon essential oil helps to prevent the spread and growth of cancer cells as well as reduce the size of tumors. One animal study showed that cinnamon extract caused cell death in tumor cells. This is how it managed to decrease growth and spread rate of the tumors.

Most of these studies that show cinnamon as being a helpful cancer fighting food have been done on animals and in test-tubes. There haven't been any studies done on humans that can prove its effectiveness on cancer cells in humans. However, it wouldn't hurt to add a teaspoon or so to your daily diet. It may be beneficial in not only preventing cancer but also decreasing inflammation, and reducing blood sugar levels.

**10: Nuts**

There have been several studies done on groups of people that could prove a link between eating nuts regularly and having a lower risk of cancer. One study followed 30,708 people for about 30 years. Every one of them was eating nuts regularly and the study found that it led to a decreased chance of contracting pancreatic, colorectal, and endometrial cancer.

Out of all the studies that have been performed, many of them have shown a positive link between nuts and their ability to prevent cancer. Brazil nuts, for example, contain a high amount of selenium. This chemical could help prevent lung cancer in people who have a low amount of selenium.

Although more studies need to be done on humans to solidify the evidence, it wouldn't hurt to add at least one serving of nuts to your daily diet.

**11: Red Grapes**

Grapes are on the list of healthy fruits you should add to your diet. Red grapes in particular carry a chemical known as superantioxidant activin which can mostly be found in their seeds. This chemical is a known cancer fighting chemical that can also be found in red wine. You can eat red grapes as a snack or eat them as regularly as you want. They can help protect against certain types of cancer as well as heart disease.

**12: Whole Grains**

Whole grains contain both fiber and antioxidants which are both proven to be cancer fighting chemicals. It wouldn't hurt to add a few whole grain foods to your diet.

## *Tips for Further Cancer Prevention*

- Wash all of your fruits and vegetables before you eat them. This will reduce the risk of eating any pesticides or other residue.
- Try eating some raw fruits and vegetables. Don't just cook everything. The raw food will have more vitamins and minerals available for your body.
- Don't cook oils or meats on high heat. Slow cooking and baking on low heat are far healthier and cancer preventing than cooking everything on a high heat. Avoid cooking anything, including meat and oil, on high heat.
- Instead of frying or sautéing your foods, try the healthier cooking options such as boiling, steaming, baking, or broiling.

- Store all of your oils in cool dark places and make sure they are in airtight containers.
- Be wary when using the microwave. Always use microwave safe containers or waxed paper when covering something in the microwave.
- Avoid anything that looks or smells like it might be moldy. It will mostly likely contain aflatoxin which is a carcinogen. It's mostly found on moldy peanuts.
- When you cook your vegetables, try only steaming them until they are tender. This will preserve as much of their vitamins and minerals as possible.

By following the correct diet and a healthy, active lifestyle, you can significantly lower your risk of contracting various types of cancer. Remember that everything is good in moderation. Even the good, healthy foods should be eaten in moderation. There is such a thing as too much of a good thing.

# Chapter 9:
# Carbs Don't Fuel Your Brain

There is a game that children like to play. I'm sure we've all played it at one point when we were younger. This game is called telephone. What this game proves is that if information is passed down through too many mouths and too many ears it gets twisted, mixed up, and changed until eventually the new information is nothing like the original information. This may be a fun and amusing game for children to play, but unfortunately it is also one of the main problems we get in the medical industry.

Information is passed from doctor to doctor, from nutritionist to nutritionist, and from patient to patient until eventually the information is turned into untrue rumors or myths that have become extremely dangerous to the public's general health. The brain fuel myth is one such instance of this happening. This myth has convinced people that the brain uses carbohydrates to fuel itself. It has encouraged people to eat a high carb diet in order to fuel their brains, but a high carb diet is unhealthy and harmful in many ways and it does not fuel our brains. This is a just another myth that has been used to line the pockets of the industry.

The brain is a very complicated thing. It's like the world's most complicated computer. It's so complicated that a human brain can't even understand a human brain. It's probably one of the most important and complicated organs in our bodies, and yet there are people out there who think they understand how it works. People like this are the reason we have such a myth as this one. Do carbohydrates fuel your brain, or are they actually bad for you? This probably looks like a simple question that should have a simple answer. However, with everyone out there fighting to be the one that knows the right answer, how can you trust any answer that is given to you?

People are now convinced that we need at least 130 grams of carbohydrates a day for our brains to function normally. This is for both adults and children. They say that if you restrict carb consumption you are effectively starving your brain. Even the largest diabetes charity organization in the world, the American Diabetes Association or ADA, says that, "The recommended dietary allowance (RDA) for digestible carbohydrates is 130 grams per day." However, none of these people actually state why we need so many carbs a day. Sure they say that the carbs fuel our brains, but where is the evidence? How do the carbs help our brains to function? No one seems to know the answer to that question. Or do they? The ADA also says, "Providing adequate glucose as the required fuel for the central nervous system." Now we have our answer! It's not 130 grams of carbs we need, its 130 grams of glucose per day that fuels our brains.

Carbs can be converted by the body into glucose, but so can fat and protein. Protein is slow and inefficient for the body to convert into glucose, so fat is probably the better choice.

## *How Does the Brain Work?*

The brain is the hungriest organ in your body. It takes up about 2 percent of your body weight, but it ends up using 50 percent of your body's glucose and about 20 percent of your body's oxygen. It's considered to be one of the more greedy organs.

When it comes to feeding your brain, it likes to burn glucose for food. It very rarely looks to anything else for fuel. Your brain spends 99 percent of your waking life operating on glucose. It's designed that way. When the brain doesn't get the glucose it needs, the results can be disastrous. If you suffer from low blood sugar or diabetes, then you've probably experienced hypoglycemia. This is what happens when your brain is starved. It results in blurry vision, slurred speech, lightheadedness, and a loss of balance. It can lead to effects far more dangerous that these as well.

The brain is designed to use only glucose as fuel. When the glucose levels in our bloodstream drop for any reason, the brain is the first organ to notice. When your brain isn't getting the amount of glucose it needs, it is literally being starved. Along with the above symptoms of a starved brain, it can also eventually lead to fatality. This is why we need glucose in our bodies and this is also why the rumor that our brains need carbohydrates has spread so far.

## *The Source of Glucose*

We know that our brains need glucose to function. What we don't know is how to efficiently get that glucose into our bodies. A study done on women in 2008 showed that women who were on a low-carbohydrate diet suffered several effects on their brains. These effects included impaired reaction time and reduced spatial memory. Women who were placed on a high-carbohydrate diet, however, did not suffer any of these effects. This research has led scientists and nutritionists to tell the public that they need to feed their bodies carbs in order to provide the right amount of glucose that their brains need.

What we aren't told is that there are other ways for your body to get what it needs. The body is like a well-oiled machine and the brain is the computer that runs it. If something is missing that is needed, the brain and body will work together to find a way to get what it needs. The same happens when the brain is in need of glucose.

There are groups of people, such as the Eskimos, who live solely on a meat-rich diet and eat little to no carbohydrates. Yet these people do not suffer any effects on their brain. The brain cannot survive without glucose. That means that the Eskimos must be getting the glucose they need from a source other than carbs.

When someone goes on a low-carb diet or one that has no carbs, their brain will quickly realize that there isn't enough glucose in the bloodstream. It doesn't take long for the situation to be solved. At this point the brain and liver will quickly work together to find another source of energy. The liver realizes it can convert other sources of food into the fuel that the brain needs. The liver can convert protein into glucose and then send it straight to the brain for immediate use. However, protein is slow and inefficient to convert, so the liver makes up for this by converting fat into something called ketone bodies and sends them up to the brain as an alternative source of energy. Your brain is able to quickly adapt to this new source of fuel and uses it as it is given.

Instead of blindly believing that our brains need carbohydrates to function, we can look at the facts and realize that what we actually need is glucose and there is more than one source for that.

### *Ketone Bodies*

Ketone bodies are a secondary fuel source for our brains when there isn't enough glucose available. It's like having a backup battery for your phone. These are backup power sources for the brain. Ketone bodies are created easily when we are on a high protein and high fat diet. These are the building blocks for our brain's backup energy source.

The reason that people aren't aware of this is because the switch from glucose to ketone bodies is not immediate. The liver can react to the lack of glucose in the body quickly but it will take a while for the brain and the body to adapt. This is why the change is usually so painful and why most people who try to go low-carb usually give up. The transition from running on glucose to running on ketone bodies is approximately 2 weeks. It takes 2 weeks for your body to fully adapt to using this alternative fuel source rather than the one it is used to. After the transition period your body and brain will not only function properly but some research shows that the brain will actually be more efficient on ketone bodies than it is on glucose.

Another advantage of the use of ketone bodies is that they last longer. Once the brain has adapted to using ketone bodies for fuel it is able to function longer on them than it could on glucose only. A brain run completely on ketone bodies can function for weeks, months, or even years on a low amount of them.

## Carbohydrates versus Fat and Protein

The Carbohydrate myth has led people to believe that they need 130 grams of carbs a day for their brains to function properly. The truth is that your body actually needs 130 grams of glucose a day. Carbohydrates are a source of glucose, but they aren't the only source. As we discussed, the body finds a way to make glucose out of protein and ketone bodies out of fat. Both of these can be used as a fuel source by our brains. We know all this, but still there is an argument as to whether we should fuel our brains with carbs or ketone bodies.

The Eskimos have proven that an all meat diet doesn't harm the brain and it actually provides them with excellent health. There is evidence to support that our brains function perfectly fine without carbs and some of our brains may even function better on a low-carb diet. There is also similar evidence that supports carbohydrates as fuel for our brains. With so much evidence supporting both low and high carbohydrate diets, it's hard to choose what is best for your own brain's functions.

When it comes to this, I guess all I can say is that the choice is up to you. The brain can function both with and without carbohydrates. All you have to decide is which diet you prefer. There are other advantages that come with a low-carb diet as well as some disadvantages. Being able to make the right choice for the health of both your body and your brain means knowing exactly what kind of life you want to live and what kind of life you can actually afford to live.

# Chapter 10:
# Viruses and Antibiotics

Recently there has been an epidemic of inappropriately prescribed antibiotics and an overuse of antibiotics as well. Most patients aren't even aware of what an antibiotic is used for or why they're being prescribed it. Along with the instances of inappropriately prescribed antibiotics, there are also instances where antibiotics aren't being used properly. All of this has led to what is called an antibiotic resistance.

## What are Antibiotics?

An antibiotic is a powerful drug that is used to treat certain illnesses. It is a very powerful medicine and can be very dangerous if used inappropriately. Antibiotics, as powerful as they are, cannot be used to treat everything. They should only be prescribed to people who have certain infections.

There are only two types of infections a person can get. Here are some examples of the two:

**Viral Infections:**

1. Colds
2. Flus
3. Sore Throats
4. Coughs and Bronchitis
5. Runny noses
6. Some ear or eye infections
7. Acute sinusitis

8. Respiratory Syncytial Virus (RSV)

**Bacterial Infections:**

1. Urinary tract infections
2. Ear infections
3. Strep throat
4. Sinus infections

Antibiotics are prescribed to people with bacterial infections and they should be used for this only. Certain antibiotics are used for certain bacterial infections. An antibiotic cannot be used to cure a viral infection. Viral infections are usually left for your body to cure by itself and an antibiotic should never be used to cure a viral infection.

In some instances a doctor won't know whether they should prescribe their patient antibiotics or not. Some viruses can cause a patient to have the same symptoms that would resemble a bacterial infection. This is where the problem comes in. The doctor can tell the patient that they have a viral infection and not prescribe them any antibiotics. However, the patient may return later after their symptoms worsen and the doctor will realize that they had a bacterial infection and they need antibiotics. At this point it may be too late to prescribe simple antibiotics as the infection could be too bad. Likewise, a doctor can diagnose their patient with a bacterial infection and prescribe them antibiotics when really they only had a viral infection. Not only do the antibiotics do nothing for the viral infection, they also cause the patient to suffer bad side effects and grow an antibiotic resistance.

## *Why Can't Antibiotics Kill Viruses?*

You can think of bacteria and viruses as types of machines. They work through all of the small, intricate parts of machinery. Viruses have a different structure than bacteria. They are two completely different machines.

Antibiotics are designed to target the part of the machinery that helps the bacteria grow. It does this so it can kill or inhibit that particular type of bacteria. It can't do the same thing with viruses because viruses are built differently and use a different type of machine to grow and replicate.

The machinery that helps the bacteria to replicate and grow is completely different than the machinery that a virus uses to replicate and grow. Therefore, because the antibiotic is designed to target the bacteria's type of machinery, it wouldn't be able to do the same to a virus's machinery. With a virus, the antibiotic won't have a target to attack.

If you try to cure a virus with an antibiotic, here is what will happen:

1. You will not cure the virus and no relief from the symptoms will be provided.
2. You won't feel better and you may even feel worse.
3. You will probably end up with some bad side effects.
4. You'll build up a resistance to antibiotics.
5. You won't prevent other people from catching your virus.
6. You'll be wasting your money and your time.

### *Antibiotic Resistance and Resistant Bacteria*

Antibiotic Resistance and Resistant Bacteria are very big issues that are beginning to arise of late. They are a big threat to global health. In fact, the US Centers for Disease Control and Prevention say that it is one of their top concerns at the moment.

Antibiotic resistance happens when a bacteria gains the ability to withstand the effects of a certain antibiotic. Basically, when once an antibiotic was used to cure a certain bacterial disease the next time it is used, it could be less effective or have no effect at all against the bacteria.

The main reason for the current rise in antibiotic resistance is the overuse of antibiotics. Antibiotics are being prescribed by doctors when they aren't needed and people aren't being properly instructed on how to use them. Another cause of antibiotic resistance comes from patients not finishing their trial of antibiotics. Patients are prescribed enough antibiotics for a certain amount of time. Sometimes they stop taking them early simply because they feel better. It doesn't matter if you feel better, your body still needs to finish the trial of antibiotics. If you don't finish all of them, then you could be adding to the bacteria's resistance to it.

There is a misconception that our bodies are becoming resistant to the antibiotics. This is just another one of those myths. Our bodies are not becoming resistant, the bacteria itself is becoming resistant.

Lately people are discussing the existence of superbugs. These are bacterial infections that have become completely resistant to any known antibiotic that we have available to us. Records state that every year at least 2 million people contract a bacterial infection that is antibiotic resistant and almost 23,000 of them die from this infection.

You're probably wondering how the bacteria are able to become resistant to our antibiotics. It does this by adapting its structure in a defensive way. It can adapt in several ways; the bacteria can learn to pump the antibiotic out of the cells. It can share its genetic material with other bacteria in order to make them resistant as well. It can neutralize the effects of the antibiotic before it is able to kill the bacteria. The resistant bacteria then survive the effects of the antibiotics and are able to spread and cause further infections. Once it spreads, the new infections are resistant to the antibiotic that was used on them or any other similar antibiotics. The only way to combat this infection is with a completely new and stronger antibiotic.

### *Don't Take Them if You Don't Need Them*

Another factor to the rising bacteria resistance epidemic, as I've already mentioned before, is the use of antibiotics when they are not needed. Some people will take an antibiotic 'just in case' if they're feeling under the weather. This is dangerous and a waste of both time and money. Taking them without needing them can also put you at risk of side effects. Some of them won't be harmful, like a rash, but some can be very harmful.

Taking antibiotics when you don't need them can also speed up the resistance to that antibiotic. This means that by the time you actually need to use them, they won't work anymore. In any case, you shouldn't have leftover antibiotics that you can take whenever.

When you're prescribed a certain amount of antibiotics, you're supposed to take all of them. If you don't finish them, even if you feel better, you don't completely kill the bacteria. A part of it is allowed to survive inside of you and that helps it become resistant to the antibiotics. Then the bacteria will come back stronger, it will hit you harder, and it will be more difficult to kill.

The best way we ourselves can combat bacterial resistance is by finishing our trial of antibiotics and by only taking them when we are told by a doctor that we actually need them.

# Curing Viral and Bacterial Infections Correctly

Using antibiotics shouldn't be that complicated, but you'd be surprised by how many people actually use them incorrectly. It's possible to forget to take them when you're supposed to. That's natural human error. However, there are plenty of other errors that people make when it comes to antibiotics when they really should know better.

Here are a few things to keep in mind when dealing with antibiotics and any kind of infection:

1. We've already discussed the fact that you have to finish your antibiotic trial. There are no if's or but's about this one. You have to finish them.

2. The antibiotics that are prescribed to you are for you only. Your doctor chose that specific antibiotic to combat your specific bacterial infection. You can't give them to someone else who has an infection. Yes, you may have the best intentions at heart but in the end you're doing more harm than good to both of you. You're given a specific amount of antibiotics for a reason. You need all of them. Even if you only give one away, that's still one that you need to take in order to fully kill the bacteria. Your bacterial infection could be completely different in structure than their bacterial infection. Even if you have the same symptoms, there is no guarantee that your antibiotics will be able to combat their specific bacterial infection. Not only will you be putting them at risk of some bad side effects, but you probably won't be helping them at all. So, whatever you do make sure you finish all of your antibiotics and never give them to someone else.

3. A cold or flu cannot be treated or cured by an antibiotic. These are viral infections and antibiotics are useless

against them. Keep in mind that a viral infection does have the ability to grow and mutate into a bacterial infection. Because of this, people often take antibiotics to try and stop the bacterial infection before it has a chance to form. This doesn't work, it will give you harmful side effects, and if your viral infection does eventually become a bacterial infection there is a high chance that bacteria will already be resistant to the antibiotic you've been taking. Don't use any antibiotics if you have a viral infection. Rather, wait until your doctor is sure it's grown into a bacterial infection and gives you the antibiotics you need.

4. A viral infection is usually left to the body to cure. You can take drugs to relieve some of the symptoms but usually all you need is rest, fluids, and some time to recover. This is the only way to cure a viral infection. Let your body do what it does best and don't mess up your health.

5. Normally, with a bacterial infection, you should just take your antibiotics as prescribed and wait. There are a few things you can do to help boost your immune system so it has a better chance at fighting the infection. Some research has shown that giving your body healthy fibers along with taking your antibiotics can help your body protect itself against the bacterial infection. The antibiotics usually attack the infection directly. The fiber can help make your body strong so it can protect itself while the antibiotics work to attack the infection.

Any other questions you have should be answered by your doctor, but it's up to you to ask the questions. Most people aren't given the information they need because they don't ask for it. If you are willing to ask the questions, your doctor will answer them.

# **Conclusion**

To conclude this book, I will leave you with one final message. Don't be afraid to take action. The problem out there is real. We are being manipulated and controlled by these big industries. Our lives have been taken out of our hands and placed in the hands of greedy businessmen. That's what the medical industry has become, a world of business and profit.

We don't have to sit down and take it. We can stand up and grab our lives right out of those greedy hands. You'll see once you start asking your doctors those hard questions they'll cave in. They'll admit they have no idea what you're talking about or they'll avoid the subject altogether just to save face. It's not only our job to ask the questions, it's also our responsibility to seek out the right answers. After all, our lives are our own and we should take responsibility for them.

You may be sitting there, marveling over everything I've told you, and you may be wondering, "What can I take away from this book?" Well that's good, because I want you to ask questions. Here is the answer:

Don't trust anything anyone tells you. Whether they're a doctor, a pharmacist, part of a weight loss and diet program, or part of the food industry. You can never fully trust anything they tell you. If they try to tell you what is what, challenge them. Ask them for more information and then take all of that information and poke holes in it. Whatever is left can be taken as a half-truth or full truth as you wish.

As I mentioned all the way at the beginning of the book, please don't take this information and use it as an excuse to forsake your doctors. They do know what they're talking about when it comes to some things and we do need them. We just don't have to fully trust them with our lives. Listen to what he has to say, just don't put all of your hope and faith into every word he says.

Not everything they say is bad for you is just bad for you. There aren't just bad calories and bad cholesterol. There are both good and bad of everything. There are good and bad calories and there are good and bad carbohydrates. The current lies and myths in the world of health will lead you to believe that you need to cut out these things altogether, but you don't. You only need to cut out the bad things and keep the good things. Your body needs calories and cholesterol, but it only needs the good kind. Keep that in mind.

Our health is under our control. We don't always have to rely on medicine and prescription drugs to maintain our body's health. We can control it through our diet and lifestyle. The things we eat can help us to lose weight, feel better, and they can even help us put off illnesses and lower our risk of cancer. We must always remember that even though sometimes medicine is needed to cure us, we can still do our part to feel better through proper diet and lifestyle.

It's good to remember there are a lot of myths out there. There's the cholesterol myth, the myth that your brain needs carbs, and of course the calorie myth. It's not just enough to know that these are myths. We need to be able to see through any other myths that we might encounter. We should always be willing to seek the truth ourselves and never just settle for what we're told. There are a lot of myths out there, some that I've told you about and some that are slowly making their way to the surface. Being able to spot a myth is a very valuable skill.

Now, I am confident that you are ready to restart your life for the better. You should be too. You've taken the necessary steps towards a better diet, and a better lifestyle. You should be proud of yourself. I promised I would lead you down the right path and here we are, at the end of the road. All that you have learned will guide you from now on. You don't need me anymore. Don't hesitate. You've started the ball rolling and you need to keep it that way. If you let the ball stop it might be more difficult to get it started again. I believe in you, but you don't need to take my word for it. All you need is to trust that you can ask the right questions and take control where you need to.

Out of all the messages there are in this book, here is the one I want you to leave with. Ask questions and take control. I've said this so many times, but that's because it is so important that you do it. You won't know all of the answers if you aren't willing to ask the questions. We are all too comfortable with other people controlling our lives, but we shouldn't be. We must take responsibility. It is the only way we can ensure that we get everything that we need out of life. This is the one thing I want you to take away from this book.

It's a big scary world out there filled with so many lies. All I can hope is that I've helped you see the truth and have led you down the right path. Soon you'll be just like me, enlightened, healthy, and living a full and free life. Let's show those big industries that they don't own us and we aren't going to let them control us anymore. Now our duty is clear: to spread the knowledge we have. Don't let your friends and family suffer like we have. Spread the truth and snuff the lies until the world is free from the greedy businessmen and we are all able to live our best lives.

# References

*11 Foods to Increase Your HDL.* (2019). *Healthline.* Retrieved 6 November 2019, from https://www.healthline.com/health/high-cholesterol/foods-to-increase-hdl#see-your-healthcare-provider

*12 Little Weight-Loss Tricks Only Nutritionists Know.* (2019). *The Healthy.* Retrieved 2 November 2019, from https://www.thehealthy.com/weight-loss/weight-loss-tricks-from-nutritionists/

*13 Foods That Could Lower Your Risk of Cancer.* (2019). *Healthline.* Retrieved 7 November 2019, from https://www.healthline.com/nutrition/cancer-fighting-foods#section6

*America.* Retrieved 7 November 2019, from https://thebreastcancercharities.org/10-cancer-causing-foods/

*Antibiotics.* (2019). Retrieved 8 November 2019, from https://www.hopkinsmedicine.org/health/wellness-and-prevention/antibiotics

*Antibiotic Resistance: The Top 10 List.* (2019). *Drugs.com.* Retrieved 8 November 2019, from https://www.drugs.com/article/antibiotic-resistance.html

Cancer, B., Cancer, C., Cancer, L., Cancer, P., Types, V., & Medicine, P. et al. (2019). *What foods and drinks are linked to cancer?. Cancer Treatment Centers of America.* Retrieved 7 November 2019, from https://www.cancercenter.com/community/blog/2017/10/what-foods-and-drinks-are-linked-to-cancer

*Cancer Prevention Diet - HelpGuide.org. (2019). HelpGuide.org.* Retrieved 7 November 2019, from https://www.helpguide.org/articles/diets/cancer-prevention-diet.htm

*Eat Less Red Meat, Scientists Said. Now Some Believe That Was Bad Advice.. (2019). Nytimes.com.* Retrieved 7 November 2019, from https://www.nytimes.com/2019/09/30/health/red-meat-heart-cancer.html

*end-point measurement. (2019). TheFreeDictionary.com.* Retrieved 2 November 2019, from https://medical-dictionary.thefreedictionary.com/end-point+measurement

Eric Metcalf, M., & Krystal Cascetta, M. (2018). *Photo Gallery: 10 Top Foods to Fight Cancer. EverydayHealth.com.* Retrieved 7 November 2019, from https://www.everydayhealth.com/cancer-photos/top-foods-to-fight-cancer.aspx

-->, <., -->, <., -->, <., -->, <., & -->, <. (2019). *Everything We Have Been Told Is A Lie - The Medical Industry Is Designed For Profit Not People! — Steemit. Steemit.com.* Retrieved 2 November 2019, from https://steemit.com/conspiracy/@jockey/everything-we-have-been-told-is-a-lie-the-medical-industry-is-designed-for-profit-not-people

*Glucose Not Carbohydrates Fuel Our Brains | HealthCentral. (2018). Healthcentral.com.* Retrieved 7 November 2019, from https://www.healthcentral.com/article/the-carbohydrate-brain-fuel-myth

guide, L., Book, U., Recipes, 2., Treats, 2., family, L., & boxes, L. et al. (2013). *The Food Pyramid - how they are wrong and why were they invented?. Ditch The Carbs.* Retrieved 2

November 2019, from
https://www.ditchthecarbs.com/why/food-pyramids/

guide, L., Book, U., Recipes, 2., Treats, 2., family, L., & boxes, L. et al. (2014). *Why high fat? Why low carb? Read all you need to know.. Ditch The Carbs.* Retrieved 2 November 2019, from https://www.ditchthecarbs.com/why/why-high-fat/

*HDL (Good), LDL (Bad) Cholesterol and Triglycerides.* (2019). *www.heart.org.* Retrieved 6 November 2019, from https://www.heart.org/en/health-topics/cholesterol/hdl-good-ldl-bad-cholesterol-and-triglycerides

*HuffPost is now a part of Verizon Media.* (2019). *Huffpost.com.* Retrieved 2 November 2019, from https://www.huffpost.com/entry/dont-trust-your-doctor_b_18977

Johnson, E., Johnson, E., Contributor, i., Garcia, A., Johnson, E., & Contributor, i. (2014). *The 10 Most Cancer Causing Foods - Breast Cancer Charities of America. iGoPink | Breast Cancer Charities of*

Khambatta, C. (2014). *Are Carbs Helping or Destroying Your Brain? | Nutrition and Fitness for Diabetes and Insulin Resistance. Nutrition and Fitness for Diabetes and Insulin Resistance.* Retrieved 7 November 2019, from https://www.mangomannutrition.com/carbs-helping-hurting-brain/

LaRosa, J. (2019). *Top 9 Things to Know About the Weight Loss Industry. Blog.marketresearch.com.* Retrieved 2 November 2019, from https://blog.marketresearch.com/u.s.-weight-loss-industry-grows-to-72-billion

*MDLinx International.* (2019). *Mdlinx.com.* Retrieved 2 November 2019, from https://www.mdlinx.com/internal-medicine/article/4008

Publishing, H. (2019). *11 foods that lower cholesterol - Harvard Health. Harvard Health.* Retrieved 6 November 2019, from https://www.health.harvard.edu/heart-health/11-foods-that-lower-cholesterol

*Red meat, processed meat and cancer | Cancer Council NSW.* (2019). *Cancer Council NSW.* Retrieved 7 November 2019, from https://www.cancercouncil.com.au/1in3cancers/lifestyle-choices-and-cancer/red-meat-processed-meat-and-cancer/

*Should You Trust Your Doctor?.* (2019). *Psychology Today.* Retrieved 2 November 2019, from https://www.psychologytoday.com/intl/blog/fighting-fear/201306/should-you-trust-your-doctor

*The 3 Lies of Fitness.* (2016). *Whole Life Challenge.* Retrieved 6 November 2019, from https://www.wholelifechallenge.com/the-3-lies-of-fitness/

*Top 10 fitness lies - busted!.* (2019). *Expertrain.com.* Retrieved 6 November 2019, from https://www.expertrain.com/blog/fitness/top-10-fitness-lies-busted.htm

*The Corruption of Evidence Based Medicine — Killing for Profit.* (2018). *Medium.* Retrieved 2 November 2019, from https://medium.com/@drjasonfung/the-corruption-of-evidence-based-medicine-killing-for-profit-41f2812b8704

*This Is the Worst Diet Advice Nutritionists Have Ever Heard.* (2019). *The Healthy.* Retrieved 2 November 2019, from https://www.thehealthy.com/nutrition/worst-diet-advice/

*What Cholesterol Means for Your Heart.* (2019). *WebMD.* Retrieved 6 November 2019, from https://www.webmd.com/cholesterol-management/features/cholesterol-bigger-picture#2

*Viral Infections - Why Don't Antibiotics Kill Viruses? - Drugs.com*. (2019). *Drugs.com*. Retrieved 8 November 2019, from https://www.drugs.com/article/antibiotics-and-viruses.html

# BENEFITS OF PLANT BASED MEDICINE

*A patients guide to plant-based medicine, essential oils and natural remedies that can treat, heal and prevent disease*

**Howard Mason**

# © Copyright 2019 - All rights reserved.

The content contained within this book may not be reproduced, duplicated or transmitted without direct written permission from the author or the publisher.

Under no circumstances will any blame or legal responsibility be held against the publisher, or author, for any damages, reparation, or monetary loss due to the information contained within this book, either directly or indirectly.

Legal Notice:

This book is copyright protected. It is only for personal use. You cannot amend, distribute, sell, use, quote or paraphrase any part, or the content within this book, without the consent of the author or publisher.

Disclaimer Notice:

Please note the information contained within this document is for educational and entertainment purposes only. All effort has been executed to present accurate, up to date, reliable, complete information. No warranties of any kind are declared or implied. Readers acknowledge that the author is not engaging in the rendering of legal, financial, medical or professional advice. The content within this book has been derived from various sources. Please consult a licensed professional before attempting any techniques outlined in this book.

By reading this document, the reader agrees that under no circumstances is the author responsible for any losses, direct or indirect, that are incurred as a result of the use of information contained within this document, including, but not limited to, errors, omissions, or inaccuracies.

# Table Of Contents

**Introduction** ................................................................ **116**
　The Side Effects of Prescription Drugs Are Silent
　Killers.................................................................................. 117
　Do Plant-Based Medicines Really Work? ....................... 119
　What You Will Learn in This Book ................................. 120

**Chapter 1: The Early Days of Medicine** ............... **122**
　Herbal Medicine and Ancient Egyptians ....................... 123
　The Effectiveness of Ancient Egyptian Herbal
　Medicine ............................................................................ 125
　Ancient Egyptian Herbal Healing Was Adopted by the
　Rest of the World.............................................................. 127

**Chapter 2: The Evolution of Medicine** ................ **130**
　The History of Pharmaceuticals...................................... 130
　The History of the FDA's Role in Modern Medicine ...... 135
　Herbal Medicine is the Enemy of the Pharmaceutical
　Industry ............................................................................. 139

**Chapter 3: Choosing Your Doctor - Why it
Matters** .................................................................. **141**
　The Difference in a DO vs. MD Doctor ..........................141
　What a Typical First-Time Visit to a DO Doctor is
　Like .................................................................................... 142
　The History of Osteopathic Medicine ........................... 143
　Treating Symptoms vs. Preventing Illness ................... 143
　The Doctor's Internal Interest in Prescribing
　Pharmaceutical Drugs ..................................................... 147
　How to Choose the Right DO Doctor for You ............... 148

**Chapter 4: The Holistic Approach** ...................... **151**
　The Holistic Doctors' Strategy ....................................... 152
　Herbal Remedies and Holistic Healing......................... 154
　Why Insurance Companies Will Not Cover Holistic
　Treatment ......................................................................... 158

**Chapter 5: Your Immune System ........................ 160**
   What is the Immune System? ......................................... 160
   The Parts of the Immune System ....................................161
   Disorders of the Immune System................................... 163
   How Processed Foods and Pharmaceutical Drugs Can Negatively Affect the Immune System ........................... 163
   How to Maintain a Healthy Immune System ................. 165
   Plant-Based Foods That Help to Boost the Function of the Immune System ................................................... 167

**Chapter 6: Cleanse and Rejuvenate Your Body .... 170**
   What is a Detox?............................................................ 170
   Reasons Why You Need to Detox ....................................171
   How Does Detoxing Work? ............................................ 172
   Benefits of Detoxing ...................................................... 172
   Common Ways of Detoxing............................................ 173
   Additional Ways to Help Your Body Detox.................... 183

**Chapter 7: Plant-Based Diet................................186**
   What are Processed Foods?............................................ 186
   What is a Plant-Based Diet? ...........................................191
   Benefits to Practicing a Plant-Based Diet ...................... 195
   How to Transition to a Plant-Based Diet ....................... 196
   7-Day Plant-Based Meal Plan......................................... 198

**Chapter 8: Essentials Oils....................................201**
   What are Essential Oils?................................................. 201
   The History of Essential Oil Use .................................... 202
   What is Aromatherapy?................................................. 203
   How Essential Oils Work................................................ 204
   Other Uses of Essential Oils ...........................................205
   Types of Essential Oils and the Part of the Plant That They Are Derived From ..................................................205
   Popular Essential Oils and Their Health Benefits ......... 209
   The Dangers of Improper Usage of Essential oils........... 210
   The Do's and Don'ts of Using Essential Oil Safely.......... 212

**Chapter 9: Herbal Medicine .................................. 214**
   What are Medicinal Plants? ............................................ 214
   Probiotics ........................................................................ 225
   List of Herbal Remedies ................................................ 228

**Chapter 10: Medicinal Garden ............................ 233**
   Benefits of Planting Your Own Medicinal Garden ......... 233
   Planning Your Garden ................................................... 235
   9 Common Herbs and Spices That You Can Grow on Your Own ....................................................................... 238

**Conclusion .............................................................. 247**
   Plant-Based Medicine Worked for Our Ancestors and It Can Work for You Too ................................................ 248
   Plant-Based Eating Can Change Your Life for the Better .............................................................................. 248
   Take Control of Your Overall Health ............................ 248

**References .............................................................. 251**

# **Introduction**

Just as plants provide us with powerful nutrition, they also provide us with powerful medicine that can treat anything from the common cold and influenza right down to cardiovascular disease, diabetes, and cancer. Headaches, diarrhea, malaria, asthma, pneumonia and tuberculosis are also common health issues that can be treated with herbal sources, and they only constitute a small portion of the long list.

Herbal or plant-based medicine is not a new concept. In fact, plants have been used medicinally for thousands of years. From the leaves and stem down to the bark and roots, plants were used to not only treat diseases, illnesses and abnormalities but also as a source of prevention.

If plants are so effective in treating so many common health issues, why are synthetic medicines being pushed down our throats, both literally and figuratively? The answer is both simple and appalling. Treating illnesses has become a big business. Pharmaceutical companies thrive on human illness and on providing temporary solutions in the form of prescription drugs. Synthetic medicines most often do not treat the root of an illness and as such the symptoms do not truly go away. The symptoms are only masked and typically recur.

Most pharmaceutical products contain ingredients derived from plants. The list of these includes aspirin, opium, quinine, and digitalis. Pharmaceutical companies have learned to capitalize on the active compounds in plants to replicate their effects temporarily.

Nothing beats what nature has provided. More than 80% of the population of developing countries depend on plants to treat medical ailments while more than 60% of the entire global population does the same. This is so not simply because plants are a cheap source of powerful relief. So many people count on herbal medicines to heal their bodies and completely change their lives because they are also accessible and plentiful. Almost anyone can plant a garden and grow common medicinal plants. In fact, many of the plants that we will discuss in this book are household names. They include chamomile, garlic, gingko, peppermint, ginger, and ginseng.

Despite the effectiveness, great availability and affordability of herbal medicine, drugs provided by pharmaceuticals are still considered a superior source of medicine by many even with the many side effects that they generate and how ineffective they often are.

# The Side Effects of Prescription Drugs Are Silent Killers

Side effects can range from mild to life-threatening. In using these prescription drugs to cure one medical problem, we often have to deal with unexpected medical problems that these drugs manifest within us.

Common 'mild' side effects that are related to the use of prescription drugs include:

- Headaches
- Dry mouth
- Diarrhea
- Dizziness
- Dermatitis or skin rashes
- Constipations
- Nausea

- Insomnia
- A general feeling of being unwell

While these are labeled as mild by pharmaceuticals and some doctors, I would say that the inconvenience and the pain they cause are far from minor. These effects disrupt daily living and can lead to more serious medical issues.

Some of the more serious side effects that can occur with the use of prescription drugs include:

- Internal bleeding
- Heart disease
- Increased blood pressure
- Liver damage
- Cancer
- Mental issues like depression and anxiety disorder, which can lead to suicidal thoughts and actions

No one knows how their bodies will react before taking a prescription drug, and the risk, which is your life, is too great to put on the line. The side effects of taking prescription drugs cannot be reversed. The sufferer has to deal with the consequences for the rest of their life, and the solution that pharmaceutical companies and some doctors offer is even more prescription drugs that can induce even more side effects. This is a vicious cycle that has to stop.

Discontinuing prescription drugs can also have negative effects on the user. Some of these drugs can cause dependency and addiction, and thus, the user will experience withdrawal symptoms after discontinued use. Withdrawal symptoms can cause sweating, shaking, nervousness, nausea, bone pain, sleep issues, depression and more.

# Do Plant-Based Medicines Really Work?

Although almost 40% of Americans have admitted to using herbal medicine to attain excellent results, there is still much skepticism toward the effectiveness of plant-based medicine. This is because plant-based medicine and supplements are not required to be FDA approved before they are made available to the public. The FDA (Food and Drug Administration) does not regulate herbal medicine because it is considered a dietary supplement rather than a drug.

However, there have been many RCTS (randomized controlled trials) that have provided evidence to support the legitimacy of the effectiveness of plant-based medicine. These tests have isolated many active compounds of several plants to show their health-related effectiveness.

One of these compounds is called capsaicin. It is the active compound in chili peppers that induces the burning sensation in the mouth when consumed. Despite what may be an unsettling sensation to some people, this compound has a long history of effectiveness in treating pain, such as low back pain, osteoarthritis, peripheral diabetic neuropathy, and postherpetic neuralgia. Qutenza is an FDA approved substance that uses chemically synthesized capsaicin to imitate the same effects.

The active compound in butterbur, a plant that is a member of the daisy family, has been shown to be a remedy for fighting pain, wounds, ulcers and inflammation. Ancient Greeks used it because of its powerful effects. It has also been synthesized to be used in migraine medications.

Green tea is another common herbal remedy. It is made so effective by its high concentration of polyphenols. Polyphenols are plant compounds that help boost brain health and improve digestion. They can be used to treat dementia, coronary artery disease, cancer, and diabetes. Their effects are so widespread that a 2015 systematic review concluded that increasing tea consumption of any kind reduces the risk of developing cardiovascular diseases such as stroke and cardiac death.

The active ingredients menthol and methyl salicylic are found in peppermint, which is a hybrid between water mint and spearmint. These active ingredients help treat a number of ailments, including irritable bowel syndrome, skin irritation, migraine headaches, tension headaches and non-ulcer dyspepsia. A 2014 study stated that peppermint oil was more effective in fighting the symptoms of irritable bowel syndrome, such as bloating, gas, diarrhea and pain, compared to a placebo. Another study in 2016 found that peppermint oil reduces the frequency and intensity of irritable bowel syndrome symptoms.

The list of evidence to support the effectiveness of plant-based medicine goes on and on.

# What You Will Learn in This Book

This book is jam-packed with insight and knowledge such as:

- The history of pharmaceuticals and how they have convinced us to live with the side effects of prescription drugs
- The history of plant-based medicines
- How to choose a doctor who truly has your best interest at heart
- How to implement a holistic approach to attacking the root of your illness instead of just treating symptoms
- How to detox your body from harmful toxins
- The benefits of detoxing

- How to implement a natural wellness plan to improve your overall health
- How to incorporate a plant-based diet in your life
- How to maintain a medicinal garden even if you have limited garden space
- So much more!

This book was written to show the harmful side effects that prescription drugs have on not only on your body and mind but on your entire life as well. It was also written to show that there is a healthier alternative that is all-natural, abundant, and cheap. That alternative is a plant-based approach to medicine and eating. My promise to you is that you will gain incredible value from every page that you read in this book. My hope is that you will use this newfound knowledge to inspire you to take a proactive approach to improve your health and wellness by the time you read the last page.

You only get one body and one life. You need to do what it takes to ensure that you treat your body with the utmost love and care. It is time to stop damaging it with the toxins left behind by prescription drugs and the consumption of processed and unhealthy foods. It is time to stop dealing with the adverse side effects gained from something that was supposed to help you and not introduce a new set of problems in your life. It is time you take a plant-based approach to not only medicine but your diet and general living. You owe it to yourself to treat your body right, and there is no better way to treat yourself than with what nature provides free of charge.

Turn the page and discover a whole new whole to illness prevention, treatment, and cures.

# Chapter 1:
# The Early Days of Medicine

The ancient Egyptian culture was a civilization that lasted from 3300 to 525 BCE. The ancient Egyptians felt that spiritual and physical health were intertwined and so they went to great lengths to ensure that physical health was maintained. The ancient Egyptians believed their gods created and controlled life through magic, demons, evil spirits, and other mythical entities. For example, some people called on the god, Serket, to heal a scorpion bite. It was thought that bad luck, disasters, and physical maladies were caused by angering the gods and dealing with evil forces. Therefore, it was not uncommon to use magic and religion to treat people. It was probably during that civilization that the concept of health began as some of the earliest records of medicine came from that period and civilization.

The healers of those times prescribed both prayer and natural remedies to patients to solve their medical problems. It is for this reason that priests were considered medical professionals. Also, there were two other types of medical practitioners, and they were magicians and healers. Magicians executed spells and charms to get rid of evil spirits that were thought to cause physical maladies. The healers were also called 'swnw.' They employed medications to cure physical ailments.

Although ancient Egyptians had limited knowledge of anatomy, they reached a level of understanding and discovery that allowed them to know that the heart pumps blood through arteries and veins to provide the body with blood. They were also aware that liver infection could cause disease even though they did not know what the specific causes were. This insight and more came from the practice of preserving deceased bodies as mummies so that the human body could be studied.

Despite the knowledge they had obtained, they were also false conceptions like a woman's uterus floated within her body and that vaginal discharge needed to be treated. Despite these false assumptions, ancient Egyptian medical practices were highly advanced for the time and included simple noninvasive surgery procedures, the setting of bones and dentistry. Their practices were so advanced that they influenced later traditions like the Greeks. In fact, by 500BC, Egyptian medicine had become so revered and respected that Egyptian healers were invited by the rulers of Rome and Babylon to visit their courts. Aspiring healers from Greece and Rome went to Egypt to become knowledgeable about these practices.

# Herbal Medicine and Ancient Egyptians

Ancient Egyptian medicine was not just about ideologies on gods and magic but also resulted from experimentation and observation. Much of this experimentation was facilitated by the mummification process, which allowed the extraction of internal organs such as the brain, lungs, liver, spleen, heart and intestines. Along with this knowledge of anatomy came the familiarization of drug preparation as plants and herbs, as aloe, cumin, fennel, castor oil, and pomegranates were used to treat illnesses and diseases. This represented the start of natural medicine. Modern scientists can study this evolution of herbal medicine from a few still-existing papyri, which are journals that were used to document the medical advances of that time.

For example, the Ebers Papyrus on ophthalmology, diseases of the digestive system, the head, the skin and specific maladies, a compilation of earlier works that contains a large number of prescriptions and recipes states that plans medicines includes cannabis, opium, henna, thyme, cassia, juniper, and linseed oil in addition to the few mentioned above. Many of these herbal remedies were soaked in wine so that they could be taken orally. This document listed 876 remedies that were made from over 500 plants.

Here are just a few of the plants ancient Egyptians used and the maladies they fought:

- Garlic. This was given to patients who suffered from bronchial and asthmatic conditions. It was also used to aid in endurance. Garlic was mashed with olive oil. This was ingested to fight the common cold. Fresh, raw garlic was also wrapped in cheesecloth or muslin and then attached to the underwear to prevent the flu and the common cold.
- Onion. This was also given to aid endurance in addition to aiding digestion.
- Cloves. They were mashed and mixed with water and vinegar to form a mixture that was gargled to treat sore throats and toothaches.
- Cumin. The seeds were considered a stimulant and were used to prevent flatulence.
- Coriander was used to treat digestive issues, as a cooling agent and as a stimulant. Both the seeds and plant were cooked in dishes to prevent flatulence. The leaves were brewed to make tea to prevent urinary tract issues like cystitis.

Medical prescriptions were written by the healers to dispense this aid. The prescription typically began with a description of the medication and was followed by ingredients and measures to be used. The method of preparation and how the final product was to be taken, whether it be as an ointment, inhaled, or by other means was included as well. This was a very sophisticated system.

## The Effectiveness of Ancient Egyptian Herbal Medicine

It is true that the ancient Egyptian medical healers did not always get it right. While injuries would be easier for them to understand and treat, diseases were a bit more difficult. This is because injuries were a clear cause-and-effect type of treatment while the causes of diseases were not always clear and so diagnosing was problematic. Therefore, ancient Egyptians thought that the cause of disease was a consequence of displeasing the gods, that the patient was under demonic attack or that the person was being haunted by a ghost. Therefore, disease was treated through the recitation of magical spells rather than with physical methods.

During the ceremony, ancient Egyptian magicians used amulets, aromas, incantations, tattoos, and more to try to drive away demons and gods and to placate the gods so that the disease could be removed. Needless to say, this was not very effective in curing or preventing popular diseases such as malaria, smallpox, pneumonia, cancer, heart disease, dementia, arthritis, high blood pressure, tuberculosis, appendicitis, kidney stones, liver disease and ovarian cysts, all of which were diseases that were common in that time.

Circumcision was a process that was also often met with failure as temple priests performed it using a flint blade as they recited incantations on boys between the ages of 10 years and 14 years. Circumcision was done to mark the boys' transition from adolescence to manhood. Unfortunately, most times this procedure resulted in infection. Since the cause of the infection was unknown to the Egyptians, it was considered the result of the influence of gods, demons and ghosts and dealt with by using magical spells. This resulted in the death of a lot of young men.

Another area that ancient Egyptians had difficulty treating was eye problems. These problems were dealt with by giving the patient a dose of bat's blood because it was thought that the ability of night vision would be transferred to the patient. Ancient Egyptian rulers also failed when dealing with female issues. Fumigation of the womb was most commonly prescribed and followed by incantations because it was believed that the womb was connected to all the parts of a woman's body. Again, this was less than effective because the cause of the problem was not treated; therefore, it persisted.

Fortunately, there were many areas that ancient Egyptians got it right apart from the use of herbal medicine to treat injuries. Healers underwent medical training to learn the profession in a school that was called the Houses of Life. This training consisted mostly of reading texts created by earlier famous healers but there did include some practical study as well.

Ancient Egyptian methods of diagnosis were so advanced that some of them are still being used today. In addition, ancient Egyptian doctors adopted an ethical code centuries before the Hippocratic Oath. The Hippocratic Oath was an inscription that stated, "Never did I do evil onto any person." Ancient Egyptian healers approached medicine in a way that kept the needs and safety of the patient as the first priority.

Dentistry was also an area that ancient Egyptians excelled. They were well aware of how to drain an abscess, how to extract teeth, and even how to make false teeth.

Ancient Egyptian healers were also knowledgeable about how to suture a word. This was done by placing raw meat upon the wound to facilitate healing and stimulate blood production. Honey was also used because ancient Egyptians were aware of its antiseptic qualities and ability to activate the presence of white blood cells, which are the chief component of the immune system. The immune system is the body's defense force against infection from dangerous invading cells such as bacteria and viruses. Even before the discovery of penicillin, ancient Egyptians healers used moldy bread as an antibiotic.

Ancient Egyptian medicine outdated both Roman and Greek medicine in both its level of knowledge and sophistication. This undoubtedly could have been attributed to the practice of embalming the dead during the mummification process. This allowed the ancient Egyptian healers to study the structure of the body and facilitated learning what parts of the body were responsible for certain tasks. Despite the limitations of the equipment and knowledge in that time, ancient Egyptians were excellent physicians. Without the results of their research and experimentation, a lot of the procedures and practices in modern medicine that have saved millions of lives would not have been possible.

## Ancient Egyptian Herbal Healing Was Adopted by the Rest of the World

The famous Greek physician called Hippocrates (450-380BC) became familiar with the herbal medicine practices of ancient Egyptians. He used this knowledge to describe 256 healing herbs. He also developed precise instructions for herb collecting and the categorization of foods and herbs by four basic qualities, which were hot, cold, damp and dry. He then theorized that disease was caused by an imbalance of the four liquids in the body of blood, yellow bile, black bile and phlegm. He stated that good health depended on keeping these in balance because they had great influence over the body and emotions.

These theories on the use of herbal medicine continued to move west and by 100 BC, the theories developed by Greek medicine had reached Rome. Around AD70, a Roman army physician called Pedanius Dioscorides described 600 medicinal herbs in his five-volume publication called De Materia Medica. This publication outlined when leaves, stems, roots, and flowers should be collected as well as when herbal remedies should be prepared. This publication had an enormous influence on medicinal practices for more than 1500 years. This influence was so significant that this was one of the first books printed after the invention of the printing press.

Around the same time, a Roman author, philosopher, and naturalist called Pliny the Elder offered a comprehensive guide that cataloged an extensive list of herbs, which were valuable as medicines. This catalog went on to become an invaluable reference for the Greek physician and philosopher called Galen (AD 130-200). Galen was the court physician to the Roman emperor Marcus Aurelius. He developed the first classification system that paired common illnesses with herbal remedies. His writings went on to become the standard for physicians of the time while the writings of Dioscorides became the standard for pharmacist of that time.

Even though the Roman Empire fell in the 5th Century, the teachings of herbal medicine moved east to Persia and Constantinople. This movement encouraged the merging of folk medicine and Egyptian traditions.

The practice of using herbal medicines continued to spread around the globe and became adopted by many more different cultures such as Arab culture, Latin culture, and through out to Europe.

Due to the invention of the Guttenberg printing press in 1440, herbal medicine writings became more popular. One such publication was written by John Gerald and was called *The*

*Herball or General History of Plants.* This was published in 1597 and was very popular because it was written in English, which meant that there was no need for knowledge of ancient languages for it to be understood.

By the turn of the 17th Century, John Parkinson published the groundbreaking works called Paradisi in Sole Paradisus Terrestris and Theatrum Botanicum, which highlighted more than 3000 plants. He was the first writer to attempt botanical classification by dividing the plants into families and classes. Many more botanists, herbalists, physicians, and astrologists went on to print works that expanded on this knowledge.

Unfortunately, it was also around the 17th Century that there was a decline in the use of herbal medicine and a shift toward the use of pharmaceutical drugs. By the 19th Century, the demand for specific drugs surged, and it seemed that many of the herbal teachings of the past were lost.

# Chapter 2:
# The Evolution of Medicine

## The History of Pharmaceuticals

Pharmaceuticals is a multi-billion-dollar industry. In fact, in the year 2017, this industry generated more than 900 billion dollars in profits and it is projected to be worth more than 1000 billion dollars by the year 2021. It is hard to believe that such a huge industry started way back in the mid-nineteenth century and gained its roots in herbal medicine.

Pharmaceuticals actually had its start by sublime traditional remedies that were big based on folk knowledge. These remedies were sold by apothecaries, who are people who prepared and soul drugs and medicines, and pharmacies. Medicine moved from the use of herbal remedies to what it is today because of the scientific revolution, which started in the 17th Century. The scientific revolution took place in Europe near the end of the Renaissance period and continued into the late 18th Century. This revolution marked the emergence of modern science and the development of subjects, such as physics, biology, astronomy, chemistry and mathematics. The advancements made at that time involved a lot of experimentation and changed the way that society viewed nature. The scientific revolution contributed Isaac Newton's 1687 Principia, the "grand synthesis" and the development of the laws of motion and universal gravitation.

The ideas of rationalism and experimentation was coupled with the idea of benefiting from human health, and this gave birth to the pharmaceutical industry as we know it today.

One of the earliest companies to move in that direction was called Merck. The German company was founded in 1668 but transitioned toward a scientific approach to medicine in 1827. The start was made by manufacturing and selling alkaloids. Alkaloids are a class of nitrogenous-based poisons and drugs. One of the most famous of them is called morphine, which is a drug that is typically prescribed to treat moderate to extreme pain. This drug works by targeting signals in the brain to change how the body feels and responds to pain.

Another early starter of the pharmaceutical industry was called GlaxoSmithKline. The company's origin was traced back to 1715, but it only started producing patented medicine in the year 1842. This company started the world's first factory for producing medicine-only products in 1859. The company's first pharmaceutical product was vitamin D, and this was released in 1924.

America was not far behind in joining the pharmaceutical revolution. In 1849, two German immigrants founded Pfizer. The founders were called Charles Pfizer and Charles Erhart. Both men were in their twenties when they started the company in Brooklyn, New York. The first product the company released was an anti-parasitic drug. While sales were moderately successful, it did not put this company on the map. That came in 1862.

Business was slow to start but rapidly expanded during the American Civil War due to the extremely high demand for antiseptics and painkillers. The company catered to demand and doubled its revenue at the start of the war.

Another huge pharmaceutical company called R&D was set up in 1876. This was founded by a former Cavalry Commander in the Union War called Colonel Eli Lilly. He was a trained pharmaceutical chemist and made a move into the pharmaceutical business after the end of his military career.

Lilly was not the only military man to get into the drug business. Edward Robinson Squibb (1819-1900) was a naval doctor during the Mexican-American war that lasted from 1846 to 1848. He used to throw drugs overboard because of the low quality, and in 1858, he set up his own laboratory. He founded the company called E. R. Squibb and Sons, which went on to become part of the modern pharmaceutical super-company called Bristol-Myers Squibb.

Other countries were not far behind to skyrocket the development of the pharmaceutical industry. Switzerland came on board in the second half of the 19th Century. The venture started with a lot of controversies because of the lack of patent laws, which led to the countries being accused of being a "pirate state." Pharmaceuticals in Switzerland started when they realize that the dyestuff they produced had antiseptic and other medicinal properties. They began to market these as medicinal products. This practice showed a clear breach of ethics because there was no differentiation between medicine and other chemicals.

Bayer was another company that initially got its roots in the dye trade. The company made the move to develop pharmaceuticals and commercialized aspirin use at the beginning of the 20th Century. It was one of the most successful pharmaceutical companies of that era. The company was so successful that it had the aspirin trademarked. At the same time, Merck bridged into the American market. In that period, pharmaceuticals were not regulated and the companies took advantage.

Insulin was made available to the market between 1918 and 1939 when Frederick Banting and his colleagues managed to isolate it. This was used to treat diabetes, which was a fatal disease until that time. The first person to benefit from the use of insulin was a 14-year-old boy named Leonard Thompson, who was dying from diabetes. The drug saved his life, and as a result, the news of insulin's effects of diabetes patients spread like wildfire. This led to Banting receiving a Nobel Prize in Medicine.

In 1928, Alexander Fleming discovered penicillin mold's antibiotic properties. Penicillin was the first modern antibiotic developed. This marked a new era for the pharmaceutical industry and its pursuit to develop drugs.

After World War II, the pharmaceutical industry gained more structure, was more regularized, and pricing schemes were introduced. The portfolio of medicinal products grew, but so did the potential ethical conflicts that arose from making money from selling healthcare products.

This lack of ethics was brought into the spotlight in 1961 with the Thalidomide scandal. This drug was marketed as a mild sleep aid and was deemed safe for even pregnant women to use. This drug caused the death of thousands of babies worldwide as it caused the development of malformed limbs.

Thalidomide was developed in the 1950s by a West German company called Chemie Grünenthal GmbH to expand its product range beyond antibiotics. The drug made users feel relaxed and sleepy, and so it was seen as the perfect alternative to tranquilizers, which were fashionable at the time. The drug was patented after testing revealed that it was nearly impossible for an overdose to occur. The testing before this patenting did not include the possible effects during pregnancy. This seemingly harmless drug was licensed in 1956 and became available without the need for a prescription in over-the-counter sales in Germany and almost all European countries. The drug helped ease the symptoms of morning sickness and so sales from pregnant women skyrocketed.

By 1960, the signs that this drug was detrimental to health started to arise. It was found that some users had nerve damage to their limbs after long-term use, and the link between the increased number of babies born with birth defects and the parent's use of the drug during pregnancy was made.

It was estimated that the death toll was over 2,000 children, and more than 10,000 children were born with serious birth defects due to the use of this drug. When taken by a pregnant mother, this drug interfered with the normal development of the baby that the mother carried within.

This scandal prompted an increase in the regulation and testing of drugs before they would be licensed for sale. In the US, there was a new amendment made to the FDA (Food and Drug Administration) rules that demanded proof of efficacy and accurate disclosure of side effects before new medications were released to the market. The Declaration of Helsinki was implemented in 1964 to put a greater ethical structure in place on clinical research so that prescribed medicines had more differentiation from other chemicals.

Since that time, many more drugs have been introduced into the market, such as the contraceptive pill, Valium, antidepressants and antipsychotics. Unfortunately, no matter the great strides made in this industry, side effects have been commonplace from the beginning, and there is no denying that these huge companies benefit from human illness.

This lack of ethics can be seen in the fact that thalidomide was still used after the huge scandal in an effort to treat leprosy, which is a chronic disease that affects the nerves, skin and mucous membranes. Signs and symptoms of leprosy include discoloration and lumps on the skin. Many patients of this disease suffer from deformities and disfigurements. This disease is caused by slow-growing bacteria and is mostly isolated to undeveloped countries such as many African countries.

This drug was placed in use in developing countries to also treat certain cancers and AIDS-related conditions even though its use still remains controversial. The risk of babies being born with thalidomide-related defects has not decreased, so this begs the question of why this drug is still being circulated for use. The answer is simple and appalling—money is being made by the pharmaceutical companies that manufacture them and the corrupt government officials in the pockets of these companies.

# The History of the FDA's Role in Modern Medicine

FDA stands for Food and Drug Administration. The US-based organization has been around for almost two centuries. The role of the FDA is to regulate about one trillion dollars' worth of products every year so that the American consumer remains safe. One of the most famous accomplishments of the FDA was its rejection of the circulation of thalidomide. The company that manufactured the drug sought approval from the FDA to sell the drug in the US in 1960, but this was rejected or when the then FDA inspector Frances Kelsey requested that the company conduct more safety studies. This move placed the FDA in a positive support light and even earned Kelsey praise from the then-US President John Kennedy. The thalidomide scandal helped pass amendments that help strengthen the FDA's drug review process.

Let's go back to where it all started in 1820 when 11 doctors set up the US Pharmacopeia to record the list of standard drugs. This was named the Food, Drug. and Insecticide Administration. This was later shortened to the Food and Drug

Administration in 1930 under an agricultural appropriations act.

It was not until 1848 that the Drug Importation Act was passed by the US Congress to require the customer service to inspect low quality drugs received from overseas. In the following years, companies were required to show proof that the drug that they provided did indeed treat the illness that they claimed.

It was not until 1906 that the original Food and Drug Act was passed by Congress. This was done on June 30th and was signed by President Theodore Roosevelt. This act outlawed States from selling and buying food, drinks, and drugs that have been tainted or mislabeled. This act allowed the FDA to get its first true victory after many decades of fighting for the government to regulate the selling and distribution of food.

The Industrial Revolution occurred in the latter half of the 18th Century and transformed rural societies of Europe and America into industrialized urban areas. It was also called the First Industrial Revolution, and the transition included moving from manual production methods to machines, chemical manufacturing and iron production. This also included the rise of mechanized factory systems and the use of steam and water power.

The Industrial Revolution introduced many consumer demands, and the opportunity for the production of food and medicine rose. As a result, both of these became large-scale enterprises. The shelf life of food was extended with the invention of canning. This allowed food to be shipped farther and to sit on shelves longer without expiring.

On the other hand, patented medicines started being sold to treat a variety of ailments. As we have seen with the medicinal industry, there was a lack of ethics that placed the consumer at a high risk. This was even true for the sale of food and drink products. There were many instances where manufacturers of food and drinks use spices and additives to mask the taste of expired meat and many other substandard ingredients. Manufacturers of patented drugs used cocaine and morphine to give consumers a high rather than actually curing their ailment. Government intervention was needed to protect consumers from this ambiguity and clear lack of ethics. This was a long and hard struggle because manufacturers had a huge influence on Congress through aggressive lobbying.

Luckily, one of the most powerful advocates for the regulation of food and drugs, Harvey Wiley, made huge strides in seeing his dream of making America medicine and food safe for the consumer a reality. He became the chief chemist at the Bureau of Chemistry in 1883 and rallied support to have the Food And Drug Act passed in 1906. His influence was so significant that the law was nicknamed the Wiley Act. He was also given regulation and power of the Bureau of Chemistry so that later amendments and laws were passed.

Unfortunately, there was a hole in this Act as it was found that it did not outlaw false medical claims but only prohibited false and misleading statements about the ingredients of a drug. This was fixed with the passing of the Sherley Amendment in 1912, which outlawed labeling medicines with fake medical claims meant to trick the consumer.

Still, the FDA recommended a total rewrite of the outdated 1906 act in 1933. The need for this rewrite was made apparent in 1957, when an inappropriately prepared medicine caused mass poisoning in the United States. This drug was called elixir sulfanilamide, and it caused the deaths of 107 people. Many of these people were children. The deaths highlighted the need to establish drug safety protocols before drugs were marketed and distributed to consumers.

This led to the passing of the Federal Food Drug and Cosmetic Act in 1938. This act required that a company prove that new drugs were safe for consumption before they were released for sale. This also led to the start of the requirement for prescription-only drugs.

Unfortunately, this was not enough to stop the death of persons at the hands of drug companies. Almost 300 people died or were injured as a result of the use of an antibiotic that was tainted with a sedative in 1941. The FDA changed manufacturing and quality protocols in response to this. This also led to the development of GMP, which stands for Good Manufacturing Practice. This is a system that ensures goods that are manufactured consistently be controlled according to quality standards to minimize the risk of pharmaceutical production that cannot be eliminated through the testing of the final product.

Again, pharmaceutical companies came under fire when an FDA nationwide investigation revealed that an antibiotic caused almost 200 deaths. This led to the FDA engaging the American Society of Hospital Pharmacies, the American Society of Medical Record Libraries, and the American Medical Association to give voluntarily reports of patient drug reactions.

Since that time, many more acts and laws have been passed that give the FDA more power to oversee consumer safety. This is enhanced by growing technology and computer usage. However, the power of the FDA is limited, and even it can't stop the ambiguity of big-name pharmaceutical companies.

# Herbal Medicine is the Enemy of the Pharmaceutical Industry

Naturally healing cannot be patented by big pharmaceutical companies. Pharmaceutical companies will not make money if you simply go out into your garden and pluck up the cure or prevention of a disease. The sad truth is that pharmaceutical companies make big bucks off of illness; therefore, it wants the global society to be sick. There would hardly be a need for prescription drugs if most people were strong, fit, and healthy.

Of the seven billion people on earth, only a small percentage are considered part of the ruling elite. This percentage controls the majority of the wealth on this planet, and of that percentage, the owners of pharmaceutical corporations have a huge seat at the table. Between the years of 2003 and 2012, the top 11 pharmaceutical companies generated almost one trillion dollars in profits.

There has been a shift away from the use of herbal medicine since the development of the pharmaceutical industry back in the 17th Century. Since that time, herbal medications have been suppressed for the use of modern medicine. Healthcare has become a big business, and its rise is dependent on human sickness. Pharmaceutical companies have a big interest in ensuring that we as a global society do not gain information or knowledge on just how effective traditional herbal medicines can be. They also have a vested interest in causing side effects that lead to the further need of drugs that they produce.

One of the most prescribed drugs are painkillers. Painkillers are highly addictive and are not only the instrumental to physical health but mental health as well. Did you know that more than 75% of the US population over 50 years of age is currently taking prescribed medication? Did you know that 25% of women in their forties and fifties have been prescribed antidepressants? Did you know that even though the US population accounts for only 5% of the global population, it consumes more than half of all prescribed drugs?

These are high figures, and they were deliberately calculated and manipulated in existence by big pharmaceutical companies. The use of prescription drugs is an epidemic that is facilitated by an army of doctors. The pharmaceutical companies control was is taught in medical schools, and your doctor may even be unknowingly playing in their hands with your health on the line. The pharmaceutical industry is a system that is rigged to keep humans chronically unhealthy in exchange for dollars.

# Chapter 3:
# Choosing Your Doctor - Why it Matters

## The Difference in a DO vs. MD Doctor

An MD doctor is one who practices allopathic medicine. Allopathic medicine refers to science-based, modern medicine. As a result, this type of doctor will regularly prescribes medication manufactured by pharmaceutical companies to treat illnesses and diseases.

On the other hand, a DO doctor is one who practices osteopathic medicine. Osteopathic medicine refers to patient treatment in a more holistic approach rather than the treatment of symptoms. This is a whole-person approach to medicine.

DO doctors are fully licensed to practice medicine and only differ in their approach to patient treatment. Both types of doctors are licensed to see patients, prescribe medication, and perform surgeries. Therefore, going to a DO doctor does not mean that a patient is compromising their healthcare

The osteopathic approach to medicine that emphasizes that the body's part all work together and influence the function of each other. This is a synergistic relationship that needs to be kept in balance. DO doctors have special training that allows them to perform osteopathic manipulative treatment (OMT). This is a group of hands-on treatment techniques that allows these types of physicians to diagnose, treat and prevent patient illness and injury. As part of a DO's education, there includes special training on the musculoskeletal system. The DO uses this knowledge to move a patient's muscles and joints using osteopathic manipulative treatment techniques that include stretching, gentle pressure, and resistance.

The benefits of OMT are numerous and can help people of all different backgrounds and ages. This treatment can be used to promote healing, increase overall mobility, and ease pain. It has been shown to be of particular benefit to people who suffer from carpal tunnel syndrome, migraines, menstrual pain, asthma, and sinus disorders.

## What a Typical First-Time Visit to a DO Doctor is Like

This includes four parts and they are:

### *The interview*

This is where a patient discusses his or her medical history with the DO doctor. Often, the patient is asked to share information about his or her work, family, and home life.

### *The exam*

The DO will perform a complete medical exam, which includes checking posture, muscles, joints, ligaments, and tendons. Tests like blood work and urine analysis will be ordered if they are necessary.

### *The diagnosis*

This is the part where the DO will consider the results of the interview and exam with input from the patient to determine what is causing the symptoms of whatever ailment it has brought the patient to the DO.

*Treatment*

The DO will suggest a treatment plan that is best for the patient and may include osteopathic manipulative treatment. Whatever course of treatment that the doctor prescribes is done to encourage the body's natural penchant toward self-healing.

## The History of Osteopathic Medicine

This approach to medicine was developed by Dr. Andrew Taylor Still in 1874. Dr. Still was inspired to develop this approach to medicine when allopathic medicine failed to save his children from dying of meningitis.

Dr. Still compared the function of the human body to a machine. He reasoned that a machine only functions at optimum when it is mechanically sound and the human body works in the same way. He believed that it is a doctor's role to improve the mechanical functioning of the human body.

Dr. Still founded the American School of Osteopathic 1892 in Kirksville, Missouri in the United States. After being open for only five years, the school had over 700 students. The doctor even encouraged women and minorities to become professional doctors.

Still and his colleague continually rallied to prove the validity of osteopathic medicine and, finally, in 1973, this persistent paid off. DOs were officially licensed to practice in all American states and were respected of equal capacity and education level as MDs.

## Treating Symptoms vs. Preventing Illness

Prevention is better than cure is the age-old saying, but pharmaceutical companies live by a different code of ethics.

The profits available from prevention are limited, while providing cures has the potential for infinite profits. Modern medicine has taught us to be reactive rather than proactive in our healthcare. We are taught to go to the doctor after we have contracted or developed an illness or disease rather than how to take preventive measures to avoid getting this disease or illness in the first place. When this disease or illness has our health hanging in the balance, then we are prescribed drugs that treat symptoms rather than curing the malady. This is how traditional medicine now works. And this is how so many people get caught in a web of continuous care from MD doctors and the pharmaceutical industry.

This is exactly why it is so important that you choose a DO doctor to provide you with measures that help prevent illness rather than treat symptoms. It is important that you place your healthcare in the hands of someone who does not have a vested interest in ensuring that you remain ill so that they make a profit.

Curing means that after medical treatment a patient no longer suffers from a particular illness or condition anymore. While there has been no progress made in finding a cure for some diseases like Hepatitis B, this is not true all around the board. In cases where the disease is not yet known to be curable, then it does make sense to seek medical treatment to manage the disease so that the symptoms do not affect the patients quality of life to an extent that life seems unbearable. However, in cases such as these, there are many herbal remedies that can aid in fighting the symptoms. Take Hepatitis B, for example. This is a viral disease that causes serious liver infection. The disease is transmitted via infected blood and symptoms can include fever, joint pain, nausea, vomiting, fatigue, and yellowing of the skin and whites of the eyes, which is a condition known as jaundice.

Normally, Hepatitis B is treated with several antiviral medications that are supposed to fight the virus while limiting the damage to the liver. But what of the possible side effects that include hair loss, stomach pain, headaches, diarrhea, sleep problems, vomiting, extreme fatigue and more? These medications are supposed to help such patients but can cause life-threatening effects instead. The use of Epivir, which is one such medication, can lead to a condition known as lactic acidosis. This condition is a buildup of lactic acid in the blood, which leads to blood poisoning and even death.

If these medications have such an extensive list of side effects that can compound the symptoms of this disease and even introduce new ones, why are not doctors telling patients about natural alternatives like milk thistle that offers relief at a much lower expense? Why aren't patients told about the long list of herbs that can help fight liver issues such as Artemisia, mistletoes, kava, nutmeg, valerian root to name just a few?

On the other hand, there are diseases that are curable yet still many patients find themselves having symptoms treated rather than the illness itself. Unfortunately, the common practice is that doctors prescribe medications to manage symptoms rather than the illness. They have been trained to do so—to treat symptoms rather than the underlying issues that perpetuate these illnesses and diseases.

This is where holistic medicine is needed. This type of medicine allows a person to seek optimal health and wellness of the entire person, meaning the body, mind, emotions and spirit. According to the holistic medicine practice, a person can only gain proper balance in life by ensuring all of these areas are performing at optimum levels. The body is made up of interdependent parts, and if one part is not working properly, all the other parts will be affected negatively. Therefore, if a person is in pain and a doctor only prescribed pain medication without looking for the underlying issue that causes the pain, then the imbalance has not been fixed and this person will not be properly healed.

Let us take a look at this example. A patient may walk into a doctor's office complaining of tension headaches. If this person visited a traditional doctor, this doctor will prescribe a medication to treat tension headaches and send the person on their way. More than likely the person will be back with the same symptoms or others because the doctor did not look into the underlying issues that were causing these headaches.

On the other hand, if the person visited a holistic doctor, this doctor would have interviewed the person to look for potential factors that are causing this person's headache. These factors of why can be wide-ranging and could be related to personal problems, stress, poor sleep habits, lack of adequate physical activity, diet and other health problems. The Do's job is to not just hand out prescriptions, but to develop a treatment plan to not only relieve symptoms but to modify the patient's lifestyle to prevent the illness, such as tension headaches, from reoccurring.

Many DO practitioners recommend that patients take responsibility for their own wellness and achieving optimum health. As a result, it is not uncommon for DOs to recommend that a patient educate themselves on making lifestyle changes to promote self-care. These lifestyle changes can include relationship and spiritual counseling, changes in diet and exercise, psychotherapy, and more. The DO may even recommend alternative therapies like homeopathy, massage therapy, acupuncture, and chiropractic care.

# The Doctor's Internal Interest in Prescribing Pharmaceutical Drugs

Many doctors get paid to prescribe pharmaceutical drugs every year. In 2015, doctors in the US alone received payments from pharmaceutical companies and companies in the medical device industry that amounted to 2.4 billion dollars. They received these payments and gifts for encouraging patience to buy pricey brand-name drugs, and this is not where the appalling statistics that show how deeply doctors are into this pharmaceutical companies ends.

Between 2014 and 2015, it was found that several doctors were paid over $25,000 during that time to prescribe opioid. Opioid is a drug with addictive properties that can lead to major psychological effects. It resembles opium and is closely related to the illegal drug called heroin. Opioid is often found in pain relievers such as oxycodone and hydrocodone, both of which are prescription drugs. The doctors who prescribe the most of these opioid prescriptions got paid the most money by these big-name pharmaceutical companies that manufacture the drugs.

This is not the only prescription drug that has been implicated in recent scandals that involve the role of doctors and their interest in the pharmaceutical industry. Doctors are routinely paid to promote pharmaceutical products. This is so severe that the Affordable Care Act was passed in 2010 and requires all pharmaceutical companies to publicly report all payments that were made to doctors that were more than $10. As a result, pharmaceutical companies have had to pay out billions of dollars to settle lawsuits because they were accused of improperly marketing and placing influence on doctors to prescribe medications to patients. More effort has been made to protect patient with the passing of the Physician Payment

Sunshine Act, which is section 6002 of the Affordable Care Act. It requires that pharmaceutical companies disclose any physician ownership or investment interest in these companies.

We go to MD doctors, we believed that they had our best interest at heart. The trust that the public has in MDs continues to crumble with the growing evidence that so many doctors are in the pockets of these big-name pharmaceutical companies. It was found in a nationwide survey in 2009 that more than 80% of doctors have some form of financial interest in pharmaceutical companies. Of this number, 20% received reimbursement for attending medical education events and meetings. That does not leave many doctors on the market that patients can trust. That is truly disheartening!

## How to Choose the Right DO Doctor for You

Your doctor is more than just someone you go to when you feel ill. This person is a confidant who can make a big difference in whether you live your life in good health or in poor condition. You certainly do not want a doctor who continuously prescribes you medication just so that he or she can make a profit by pushing the drugs that pharmaceutical companies design and manufacture down your throat both literally and figuratively.

Here are a few tips you can use to choose the right health care provider for you:

- Ask around for good DO doctors. DO doctors do not have the vested interest in pharmaceutical companies that many MDs do. DO doctors are less likely to prescribe medications, especially pricing medications that just deal with symptoms. These kinds of doctors were taught to treat the whole person, and therefore, focus on how the person can improve their lifestyle to maintain good health.

- Ensure that this doctor is in a convenient location. I am sure that you will not want to travel very far if you are not feeling well to see your doctor. Therefore, ensure that your doctor's office is conveniently located to suit your needs.

- Perform a quality check. Do your research before you go to any doctor. In this day and age, it is simple enough to get on the internet to check on reviews on a doctor. You can even find out if this person keeps up-to-date in the latest developments in the medical field with updated certification.

- Do a cold call. You can tell a lot about a doctor ethic and approach to medicine by phone etiquette of the office staff.

- Keep your needs in mind before you visit any doctor. If you are reading this book then I can assume that you would like a holistic approach to your healthcare. Keep that in mind when you visit the doctor so that you are not swayed in another direction and get placed under the thumb of a doctor's greedy intentions.

- Learn to listen to your gut. We form opinions about other people within seconds of meeting them, but we have been taught to stifle this intuition. Listen to your inner voice, and check to see if your feel at ease with this doctor. Watch how this person behaves. Is he or she kind to his staff and to other patients? Does he or she answer your question and explain things in a way that you clearly understand? Does this person make a concerted effort to listen to your difficulties and concerns? You need to be able to trust your doctor and to talk comfortably with this person. Usually, your gut can tell you whether or not you can trust this person.

# Chapter 4:
# The Holistic Approach

Holistic healing has many stereotypes attached to it. Some people see it as voodoo and magical nonsense that has no sound foundation. However, that is far from the truth. The true definition of holistic healing is the characteristic of comprehending that the human body houses several parts that are intimately interconnected to create a whole body. The whole body functions best when there is synergy between these interrelated parts.

Holistic healing is not just an approach to healthcare. It is an entire lifestyle because your health is not just your body. Your health encompasses your mind and your soul as well. You cannot transform one without transforming the others. Holistic healing is dependent on education so that a person can maintain or restore balance of the mind, body, and soul so that the entire individual can function as a well-maintained and healthy whole.

It is because the ancient Egyptians and the civilizations that came after them recognized the importance of keeping these interconnected parts working in balance that there were such huge strides made in the development of herbal healing. Even Hippocrates was known to promote the power of self-healing. He not only believed that the body had the capability of healing itself from most diseases, but he also encouraged it. Unfortunately, these holistic practices were stifled under the rise of the pharmaceutical industry.

Luckily, this is not an indefinite state of affairs. We as a global society have the power to reclaim control of our bodies and strengthen the body's capabilities to heal itself with what nature has provided us.

Herbal medicine is an essential part of a holistic lifestyle. In this one instance, reliving the past and the way our ancestors approached healthcare can be the way for uplifting the future so that we are healthier and happier.

You can use the engine properties of holistic healing to benefit yourself and become healthier. There are immediate and long-term benefits to exploring this ancient way of healing. Holistic doctors are showing more and more patients how they can challenge the body to open up the mind and spirit so that they can engage their mind for a more fulfilling life. With the guidance of a holistic doctor, you can obtain good life and health for yourself too.

## The Holistic Doctors' Strategy

DOs are just one type of holistic medical practitioner. There are others including integrative physicians, who use a blend of holistic and mainstream medicine; ayurvedic doctors, who use life energy to govern medical practice; and naturopathic doctors, who encourage the body's self-healing abilities to become more prominent. No matter which of these doctors you choose, they all encourage holistic healing practices. All of these doctors promote the attack of the root cause of illness instead of just treating the symptoms. They also aim for preventative medicine and improving overall health.

Holistic medicine also goes by the name of alternative medicine. By Western standards, the advice and healing obtained from alternative medicine is considered untraditional. Despite what is considered the unconventional approach, there is no denying that an increasing number of Americans are finding relief from the illnesses when using the methods prescribed by holistic doctors. Here are a few common alternative medicine techniques that are encouraged by these types of doctors:

- Acupuncture. This is a treatment method with origins in China. This practice is based on the belief that blocked energy centers in the body cause illness and sickness. Thin needles are inserted into specific points on the body by a licensed practitioner to relieve this blockage. Many people who suffer from chronic headaches, chronic back and neck pain, and osteoarthritis have found relief with this technique.

- Chiropractic. This is practice by chiropractors who are licensed doctors trained in spinal adjustment. This has been shown to offer relief from neck pain and headaches.

- Homeopathy. This technique is based on the principle that whatever is causing an illness can be used to treat it. Therefore, practitioners of this method will take a substance that is known to cause harm and dilute it to a near vanishing point to treat an illness. This technique should be approached with extreme caution.

- Meditation. This technique has been used by many people who suffer from mental illnesses, such as anxiety and depression, those who suffer from insomnia and even those who suffer from irritable bowel syndrome. The technique focuses on using deep breathing to center a person to help the mind heal the body from the inside out.

- Massage. Massages are not just great for relaxing but also help with relieving several types of pain, including back pain and pain from injuries.

- Yoga. This is an ancient practice, and it has been around for so long because it has several health benefits, which include reducing blood pressure, easing depression, and relieving lower back pain.

- The use of foods to cure the body. You are what you eat; therefore, holistic doctors encouraged the consumption of healthy and clean foods so that the body becomes clean and healthy. Several foods that are encouraged for consumption include berries for its anti-inflammatory and antioxidant properties; and apple cider vinegar, which helps reduce the risk of cancer, promotes weight loss, help regulate blood sugar and aids in lowering bad cholesterol. Teas and turmeric are common recommendations as well.

- The use of probiotics. Probiotics are the good bacteria in the gut of every human. They not only aid keeping a good balance in the digestive system but also help in maintaining overall health.

- Herbal medicines. Many holistic practices are governed by the fact that the body has several natural self-healing abilities. Holistic doctors work to encourage these abilities to perform better with the air of herbal supplements such as feverfew, which has been shown to decrease the frequency of migraines in some patients, and saw palmetto, which can be used to treat the symptoms of an enlarged prostate.

Other alternative medicine practices include aromatherapy, tai chi, reiki, progressive relaxation, guided imagery, cold water therapy, and hypnotherapy.

# Herbal Remedies and Holistic Healing

Herbal medicine is also called phytomedicine, and its ancient roots have shown us that we can use a plant's flowers, bark, leaves, fruit and roots for medical purposes. The use of herbal medicines can promote the balance of body, mind, and soul and can enhance vitality, promote longevity, and enhance overall health. Herbal medicine has the power to cure, treat, and prevent a wide range of illnesses and diseases from common to rare types. Not only are the benefits far-reaching, but the variety of goods available are astounding. There is a list of several herbs that can aid in maintaining and restoring your overall health. They are listed by the condition that they treat.

## *Anxiety*

This is a mental disorder that is characterized by a general feeling of unease, such as worry or fear. The feelings can range from mild to severe and can affect anyone of any age. There are a few room herbal remedies that can aid in soothing these extreme feelings. They include ashwagandha, lavender, lemon balm, passion fruit, St John's wort, valerian, chamomile and kava kava, which is a plant that is commonly found in the Pacific Islands.

## *Depression*

This is another mental disorder. It is characterized by feelings of dejection and severe sadness. The following herbs can aid in uplift the spirits of those who suffer from this disorder. They include St. John's wort, ginseng, chamomile, lavender, and saffron.

## *High blood pressure*

This is also known as hypertension, and it occurs when the body's blood pressure increases to an unhealthy level. This is calculated by measuring how much blood is passing through blood vessels and the amount of resistance that the blood meets when the heart pumps. Herbal remedies that can aid in reducing hypertension include flaxseed, ginger, garlic, celery seed, basil, cinnamon, cardamom, and cat's claw.

## Migraines

These are characterized by pulsing, throbbing and excruciating pain around the head, neck, and face. The pain can be debilitating. There are herbal remedies that can provide relief. They include ginger, feverfew, coriander seeds, raw potato cuttings, horseradish, yarrow, willow, valerian, rosemary, and lavender.

## Kidney stones

Kidney stones are hard deposits that form in the kidneys. These hard deposits travel through the urinary tract and can cause extreme pain when they exit the body. Herbal remedies that can provide relief include celery seed, wheatgrass, basil, pomegranate, and dandelion.

## High cholesterol

The body does need cholesterol to function optimally; however, there are two types of cholesterol. The good type of cholesterol is known as HDL (high-density lipoprotein) cholesterol, and the bad type of cholesterol is known as LDL (low-density lipoprotein) cholesterol. To keep levels of LDL cholesterol down, the recommended herbal remedies include flaxseed, garlic, hawthorn, green tea, coriander seeds, fenugreek seeds, psyllium husk, and amla.

## Heartburn and acid reflux

Millions of people worldwide suffer from these two conditions, and there are a few herbal remedies that can help in treating the symptoms. They include chamomile, lemon balm, caraway, licorice, peppermint, angelica, and milk thistle.

## Hernia

A hernia is a condition that occurs when an organ pushes through the organ tissue or muscle that holds it in place.

Herbal remedies that can correct this include aloe vera and chamomile.

## Boosting libido

A low sex drive can affect many aspects of a person's life. Luckily, there are herbal remedies, such as the consumption of bananas, figs, and avocados to boost libido. Herbs and other herbal remedies that aid in boosting libido also include ginkgo, ginseng, maca, tribulus terrestris, saffron, fenugreek, and saw palmetto.

## Sore throat

We all know the discomfort and inconvenience of having a sore throat. Luckily, there are herbal remedies that can ease the pain in a shorter period. They include licorice, lemon, ginger, sage, Echinacea, fenugreek, peppermint, and chamomile.

## Common cold and flu

Just like a sore throat, this can be highly inconvenient and uncomfortable to deal with. However, ginger, garlic, and Echinacea are just a few of the herbal remedies that you can use to get the symptoms under control.

## Constipation

If you have a hard time going, try using herbal remedies such as Senna, peppermint, Ginger, dandelion, black or green tea, licorice, or chamomile.

## Menstrual cramps

Turmeric, chaste berry, and black cohosh are just a few of the effective home remedies that can help alleviate the pain of menstruation.

## Menopause

Herbal remedies such as red clover, dong quai, ginseng, and evening primrose can help give relief of menopausal symptoms.

## Congestion

Using herbal remedies such as chamomile, green tea, and garlic can clear your nasal passages quickly.

As we go farther into this book, we will touch on some of these herbal remedies in more depth and other ailments that can be cured and prevented with the use of herbal remedies. We will also touch on how a holistic approach to healing can aid in strengthening the immune system, balance hormones, and more.

# Why Insurance Companies Will Not Cover Holistic Treatment

Consumer demand for alternative sources of medicine is at an all-time high, yet there is a resistant to providing patients with insurance coverage when they use natural medicine.

The United States has an expense of 1.5 trillion dollars on healthcare annually, even though most Americans are not satisfied with the healthcare system. This dissatisfaction is why many turn to alternative and natural sources of medicine. Unfortunately, these people have been forced to place their hands in their own pockets to supplement the cost of pursuing a natural medicine to improve their health.

Only a few strides have been made in having insurance companies cover alternative medicine. This includes coverage for chiropractic and acupuncture visits. Almost all other natural treatments are excluded from insurance coverage. This begs the question of why there is a hold up in adding natural medicine coverage to insurance plans, especially when holistic doctors follow the same steps that conventional doctors use.

The answer is obvious. Just as with most other things in the world of medicine, the pharmaceutical industry is causing the stall on this. Pharmaceutical companies do not want to encourage any use of natural medicine, as this will cut into their profits. It is sad to realize, but pharmaceutical companies extend influence even over health insurance. When asked why they do not cover natural medicine, many health companies will say that there is not enough evidence to prove the effectiveness of natural medicine even after centuries of proof has been provided. Insurance companies claim that they do not want to take on the risk of supporting a medicine that has not been proven as a form of treatment. Simply put, they do not want to pay for a treatment that they are not sure is valid. The plain truth is that unhealthy and ill people pay more in insurance because they expect the worst.

Insurance companies have a vested interest in keeping you sick as well. A lot less people would not carry insurance if they did not foresee major illness in their future.

It is clear to see that we as a global society cannot depend on the pharmaceutical industry or even health insurance companies to watch out for our best interests. We have to take on that responsibility ourselves. Educating yourself is the first step to taking that power back from these big-name companies. This book can help you to nourish your mind with the facts so that you can achieve that whole body balance.

# Chapter 5:
# Your Immune System

## What is the Immune System?

The immune system is a complex network made up of organs, tissues, and cells that fight infections from bacteria, viruses, parasites and fungi, and set up systems to deal with infections should they manage to occur. The immune system is the body's natural defense system against cells that are bad for it.

These invaders can come from several sources, such as breathing in these invasive cells, ingesting contaminated food or water, or through physical contact, such as touching skin or having sex, and even through the eyes. These invasive cells can also get into the body through shared needles and insect bites.

The immune system uses several lines of defense to block out these invaders. Such defensive measures include:

- The skin, which is a waterproof barrier that secretes oil and contains cell properties that suppress and kill invasive cells.

- The digestive tract, which is lined with a mucous layer that contains more of these cells and properties. The digestive tract also contains acid in the stomach, which can kill invasive cells as well.

- The lungs, which are lined with a mucous layer to trap foreign entities. This mucus layer is moved upward by small hair-like structures so that it can be coughed out to remove any trapped invasive species.

- Saliva and tears contain antibacterial enzymes that help reduce the risk of foreign entities entering the body.

These are only a few of the defenses that the body has in place to keep harmful invasive species away.

The body is good at preventing repeated infections when these invasive species do manage to get through by remembering the properties of these invasive species so that it can be ready to defend the body faster the next time. This is facilitated by special cells known as memory cells that recognize and destroy microbes quickly when they enter the body again. The invasive infections knowns as the flu and common cold change the makeup of their cells often, which is why human beings have a hard time preventing the contraction of these infections.

# The Parts of the Immune System

The immune system is made up of several parts. They include:

- White blood cells. These are manufactured in the bone marrow and are part of the lymphatic system. They travel throughout the body through the blood and tissues looking for invasive cells so that they can launch an immune attack when the find these invaders. There are several types of white blood cells.
- Antibodies. Antibodies are crucial to the immune defense of the body. They recognize substances that are called antigens on the surface of microbes, or the chemicals that the microbes produce that mark them as foreign to the body. When the cells recognize these antigens, they mark the cells for destruction and as such as cells, proteins, and other chemicals move in for this attack.

- The complement system. This system is made up of special proteins that work in conjunction with antibodies to mark and destroy foreign entities.

- The lymphatic system. This is a complex system made up of delicate tubes that run throughout the body. The system is made up of lymph nodes that trap foreign entities; lymph vessels that are tubes that carry lymph, a colorless liquid that bathes the body tissues and contains white blood cells; and white blood cells, which are also called lymphocytes. The lymphatic system aids the immune system by managing the fluid levels throughout the body, reacting to the presence of foreign entities, locating and destroying cancerous cells, locating and destroying cell products that can lead to diseases or disorders, and absorbing some of the fat from our diets from the intestines.

- The bone marrow. This is a spongy tissue that is found inside of our bodies. It manufactures several cells, including the red blood cells that are needed to carry oxygen throughout the body; the white blood cells that are used to fight infection; and platelets, which we need for our blood to clot in the event that we sustain an injury.

- The spleen. This organ is responsible for blood filtering and aids in the removal of foreign cells in addition to destroying old or damaged red blood cells. It is also responsible for making components like antibodies and lymphocytes.

- Thymus. This aids in producing white blood cells called T-lymphocytes and also monitors and filters blood content.

# Disorders of the Immune System

Sometimes the function of the immune system can be exaggerated beyond what is needed. One such exaggeration includes allergic reactions and diseases. Allergic reactions are defenses the immune system uses in response to allergens that are overly strong. These include allergies to medication, food, and insect bites. Another such example is known as anaphylaxis, a severe allergic reaction that can lead to death in response to throat or tongue swelling, shortness of breath, lightheadedness, vomiting and low blood pressure. Examples of overreactions of the immune system include asthma, hives, dermatitis, eczema, sinus disease, and hay fever.

Another example of over-activity of the immune system is autoimmune diseases. Such diseases include type 1 diabetes, rheumatoid arthritis, and multiple sclerosis. Autoimmune diseases arise when the immune system mounts a defense against normal functions of the body.

The immune system can also underreact in a condition called immunodeficiency. This under-activity makes people vulnerable to infections that can be life-threatening. Immunodeficiency can arise due to genetics, medical treatment such as the use of pharmaceutical drugs, such as corticosteroids and chemotherapy, or be caused by other diseases, such as HIV/AIDS.

# How Processed Foods and Pharmaceutical Drugs Can Negatively Affect the Immune System

As the saying goes, "You are what you eat" and this applies to your immune system. Consuming a lot of processed food can sabotage your immune system. The first reason this can occur is because consuming too many processed foods can lead to poor gut health. There is a delicate balance of good and bad bacteria living in your digestive system. The good bacteria break down food, aid in the absorption of nutrients, and help keep toxic materials out of your body. These good bacteria rely on a good supply of vitamins and minerals to keep them in good working order. Consuming the huge supply of sugar, salt, and unhealthy fats that are obtained in processed food throws off the fine balance of this entire ecosystem.

This allows the growth of bad bacteria and yeast, which overpowers the presence of good bacteria. This compromises the function of the immune system not only because these microbes are already present in the body but also because the function of keeping other microbes out of the body is compromised. The only way to avoid these issues is to drastically reduce the consumption of processed foods so that you can eliminate toxins from your diet. They should be replaced with healthy options that provide the body with healthy nutrition and the probiotics it needs to maintain the healthy balance of microbes in the gut.

Secondly, consuming processed food increases inflammation in the body. This arises as a response from the immune system to deal with the consumption of too much sugar, salt, and unhealthy fats. The more the body is bombarded with processed food, the more the immune system overreacts and increases inflammation. Chronic inflammation can impair the function of the immune system severely.

This can be reversed by consuming less processed foods and consuming more anti-inflammatory foods, such as tomatoes, olive oil, fruits, nuts, green leafy vegetables and fish, such as salmon and tuna.

The immune system is not only weakened by the consumption of processed foods but possibly by the pharmaceutical drugs that you take. Some pharmaceutical medications contain a dangerous side effect, which is weakening of the immune system. This places you at risk of developing several infections, all in the name of fighting off one illness. These are called immunosuppressant drugs. There are several types of immunosuppressant drugs and they include:

- Corticosteroids. These are typically used to provide relief from inflammation in certain parts of the body. Popular types include prednisone, Deltasone and Orasone, budesonide, and prednisolone.
- Janus kinase inhibitors. These are a type of drug that works by inhibiting the activities of certain hormones that are needed to facilitate the function of the immune system. An example is tofacitinib.
- IMDH inhibitors. These suppress the synthesis of adhesive reception that are needed to regulate cell-to-cell contact. This can inhibit the role of white blood cells and antibodies. Examples include azathioprine, leflunomide, and mycophenolate.

Other drugs that inhibit the functions of the immune system are biologics, mTOR inhibitors, TNF inhibitors, and calcineurin inhibitors.

It is ironic that doctors prescribe these medications in a bid to help you become healthier, but these same medications put you are risk for infections that can impair your health more.

# How to Maintain a Healthy Immune System

Now that we have established how important the immune system is to good health, here are a few ways you can ensure that yours remains strong:

- Ensure that you are getting enough sleep. Getting the right amount and good quality sleep is as essential to maintaining a healthy body as eating and breathing are. Adults typically requires seven to nine hours of sleep nightly to reap several health benefits, one of which is a strengthened immune system.

- Eat less sugar. Consuming sugars slows down the function of the immune system; therefore, its attack to fighting foreign entities. Substitute sugar for healthier alternatives such as plant-based stevia and maple syrup.

- Practice deep breathing techniques. We breathe unconsciously, but the impact that breathing has on our overall health is great. Getting enough oxygen fuels you with energy and a lack of proper supply contributes to many health issues such as the development of cancer, heart disease, digestive problems, aching joints, and respiratory problems.

- Eat more fermented food. Examples of fermented foods include miso, kimchi, tempeh, sauerkraut, and yogurt. Fermented foods contain enzymes and probiotics that are not only aid in improving the function of the digestive system but also strengthening the immune system.

- Spend more time outdoors. Spending time basking in the sun provides your body with the much-needed Vitamin D, which plays a vital role in supporting the immune system.

- Do a detox diet. Unfortunately, we live in a world that is filled with pollution and many individuals consume substances that introduce toxins into their bodies on a daily basis. These substances include caffeine, sugar, alcohol, gluten, dairy, and the chemicals found in processed foods. A detox diet aids in removing these toxins from the body by promoting the consumption of whole grains, vegetables, and fruits. In addition to removing toxins from the body, these foods provide needed nutrition that aids in strengthening the immune system.

- Practice stress relieving techniques. Stress suppresses the function of a healthy immune system. Laugh more, practice yoga, meditate and find other ways of enjoying life so that your immune system can work better.

- Increase your antioxidant intake. Antioxidants help strengthen the immune system so consuming more antioxidant-rich foods and drinks such as dark chocolate, blueberries, and green tea should be a priority.

## Plant-Based Foods That Help to Boost the Function of the Immune System

The way that you eat determines whether your immune system is strong or weakened. Here are a few fruits and vegetables that you can consume to strengthen your immune system:

- Citrus fruits. There is a long list of citrus fruits, and this list includes oranges, tangerines, lemons, limes and grapefruits. These foods are rich in vitamin C, and vitamin C increases the production of white blood cells, which is key for fighting off infections and boosting the function of the immune system. Unfortunately, the body does not store or produce vitamin C so continuous consumption is required to ensure that levels remain at optimum.

- Red bell peppers. These contain twice as much vitamin C as citrus fruits. They also contain beta carotene, which helps to keep your skin and eyes healthy.

- Garlic. Garlic contains heavy concentration of sulfur-rich compounds that aid in strengthening the immune system. Garlic also helps lower blood pressure and slow down the hardening of blood arteries.

- Ginger. Ginger is a food that you can use in the aftermath of an infection, such as the common cold or the flu to help decrease inflammation, soothe a sore throat, and decrease nausea.

- Broccoli. This food is packed with vitamins, minerals, fiber, and antioxidants. Ensure that it is cooked as little as possible to reap the most benefit.

- Spinach. This is packed with beta carotene, vitamin C, and antioxidants. Again, this is a vegetable that should be cooked as little as possible to get the most nutritional value from it.

- Green and black tea. Both of these teas are rich in flavonoids, which are a type of antioxidant. Green tea is also a good source of an amino acid called L-theanine. This amino acid is needed for the production of lymphocytes.

- Papaya. This fruit is loaded with vitamin C and also has a digestive enzyme called papain, which has anti-inflammatory properties.

- Kiwi. This contains high levels of vitamin C.

- Sunflower seeds. These contain several vitamins and minerals, one of which is vitamin E, which is a powerful antioxidant.

- Avocado. This contains high levels of vitamin E.

- Dark green leafy. They also contain high levels of vitamin E.
- Almonds. This is another food that contains high levels of vitamin E.

# Chapter 6:
# Cleanse and Rejuvenate Your Body

We live in a world that is filled with pollution. It is in our food, in the air that we breathe, the things that we touch, and more. Our bodies were designed to naturally detoxify and remove these toxins but with such a high level of pollution, our bodies can become overburdened easily and needs help in the detoxification process.

Detoxification has been used for centuries by different cultures around the world to maintain and renew optimum health, to feed the body, to maintain health and nutrition and to protect the body from disease. These past centuries of knowledge can help you achieve the same for your body.

## What is a Detox?

This is a short-term diet intervention designed to eliminate toxins from the body. There are several ways to detoxify the body, and we will discuss a few common methods below. But first let's take a moment to speak on what a detox does for the body. A detox:

- Helps improve blood circulation
- Provides the body with healthy nutrition
- Stimulates the liver to get rid of toxins
- Helps restore the body organs
- Promotes the elimination of toxins through sweat urine and feces

# Reasons Why You Need to Detox

Not sure if you need a detox? Here are a few signs that your body may be giving you that it is crying out for one:

- You often feel lacking in energy, fatigued, and a general feeling of being unwell. A detox diet is said to help you feel more alive, happy, and full of energy because it is the presence of these toxins that often has a person feeling brain fog, body achiness, digestive issues, headaches, allergies, and other issues that generally bring us down.

- You often suffer from sugar and carb cravings. Carbohydrates are used by the body to generate energy. Sugars are the simplest form of carbohydrates. Initially when carbohydrates are consumed, we experience a rush of energy that makes us feel invincible at times but soon after we experienced an energy crash. Unfortunately, when we consume sugar, it stimulates the reward center of our brains, which makes us crave more sugar to get over the sugar crash. The stimulation of the reward center of the brain by sugar makes it an addictive substance. Excessive sugar intake leads to several negative health benefits, including obesity, the development of cardiovascular diseases, type 2 diabetes, kidney and liver problems, and more

- You suffer from issues of weight loss. If you cannot lose weight and keep it off, this may be a sign that your body is in need of a diet to get rid of toxins in addition to eating healthier. Most of the weight loss management issues we have arise because we practice a diet that is rich in processed foods that carry empty calories and do not have the nutrition that our bodies need. This can lead to weight gain. In addition, these processed foods are often high in sugar, which is an addictive substance. Excessive sugar intake triggers insulin spikes and inflammation, both of which are conditions that make it hard to maintain a healthy weight.

Other reasons include:

- You have never detoxed. Detoxifying should be done at least once a year.
- You often suffer from allergies
- You often suffer from low-grade infection
- You are often bloated
- You suffer from menstrual problems
- You often suffer from irritated skin
- You often feel mentally confused
- You have puffy eyes or bags underneath the eyes

## How Does Detoxing Work?

Detoxifying sounds like a complicated process, when in actuality it is quite simple. The process of detoxification removes impurities in the blood by delivering them to the liver where they are processed for elimination. These toxins can also be eliminated through the lungs, intestines, kidneys, lymphatic system, and skin. The body has systems in place to deal with impurities and toxins, but when they are not properly filtered, the body is adversely affected. This is why detoxifying is such a valuable process to partake in.

## Benefits of Detoxing

Detoxification is an important component of maintaining optimum health, and here are just a few benefits that you will be rewarded with when you detoxify your body:

- Reduced inflammation
- Healthier and improved appearance of skin
- Healthier Fuller hair
- Strengthened immune system
- Boosted energy levels
- Better weight management
- Improved performance of digestive system
- Better smelling breath
- Improved mood and mental health
- Improved focus and concentration
- Increased longevity

# Common Ways of Detoxing

### The Smoothie Cleanse Detox Diet

This detox diet is based on replacing the regular meals of breakfast, lunch, and dinner with nutritionally balanced smoothies made from whole plant-based ingredients. This detox diet follows the following rules:

- There is to be no consumption of seafood, cheese, meat, processed foods, alcohol, or bread.
- Three smoothies shall be consumed daily with two snacks in between.
- At least 12 glasses of water should be drank daily.
- 30+ minutes of physical exercise is required daily.
- This diet should be practiced for at least five days.

### Easy Detoxifying Smoothie Recipes

To help get you started on your smoothie cleanse, here are a few ingredients mixes that you can use. All you need is a blender. Throw in the ingredients and blend until a smooth, uniform consistency is attained. To ensure that your smoothie has balanced nutrition, here are a few guidelines to follow:

- Add at least one handful of green leafy vegetables such as spinach, kale, or bok choy.
- Ensure that you get your fiber by adding oats, chia seeds, or flax seeds.
- Add healthy fats like avocado, nut butters, or coconut oil or butter
- Obtain your protein requirement by adding protein powder, Greek yogurt or nut butters.
- Liquid bases such as coconut milk, almond milk, and unsweetened fruit juice can be added.
- Use water or ice to smoothen out the smoothie without adding calories.
- Honey or maple syrup can be used as a natural sweetener, but ingredients such as yogurt, fruit, and nut butter are already sweetened so you may not need to add a sweetener.

Without further ado, here are the ingredient list for tasty smoothies that can be prepared in five minutes or less and are one serving.

**Almond Zucchini Smoothie**

- 1 yellow zucchini, chopped
- 2 tablespoons of almond butter
- 1 pear
- 1 cup of almond milk
- 1 cup of spinach

- 1/2 teaspoon of cinnamon
- 1/2 cup of water

**Berry Spinach Smoothie**

- 1 cup of mixed berries
- 3 tablespoons of almond butter
- 1 cup of almond milk
- 3 tablespoons of Greek yogurt
- 2 stalks kale with the ends chopped off
- 1/2 teaspoon of honey
- 3 tablespoons of chia seeds

**Green Grapefruit Smoothie**

- 1 cup spinach
- 1/2 avocado
- 1/2 tablespoon of grated Ginger
- 1 cup of chilled green tea
- 1 small banana
- 1 scoop vanilla protein powder
- 1/2 tablespoon of lime juice

**Ginger Carrot Smoothie**

- 1 large carrot, chopped
- 1 tablespoon of grated Ginger
- 1/2 teaspoon of turmeric powder
- 1 chopped pear
- 2 kale stalks with the ends dropped off
- 1 tablespoon of coconut oil

- 1 tablespoon of flax seeds
- 1 cup of ice

**Matcha Almond Smoothie**

- 1 teaspoon of matcha powder
- 4 tablespoon of almond butter
- 1 cup spinach
- 1 avocado
- 1 pear
- 1/2 teaspoon of vanilla extract
- 1 cup of almond milk

**Snacking on the Smoothie Cleanse Detox Diet**

When snacking on this detox diet, snacks should be limited to 200 calories or less. To keep things interesting, you can have a different snack every time. Some great snack options include:

- Seeds and nuts
- Veggie chips
- Dehydrogenated fruit
- Chopped veggies with guacamole or nut butters such as almond butter, peanut butter and cashew butter
- Greek yogurt
- Granola

*The Simple Fruit and Veggie Detox*

This detox diet promotes the consumption of fruits and vegetables only for three days. This detox plan is particularly attractive to people who would like to lose weight fast and conquer food addiction quickly. The basic rules are:

- Drink at least 12 glasses of water every day
- Do not drink any non-water beverages including tea and coffee
- Eat only fresh fruits that are preferably organic. No canned, frozen, or dried fruits allowed.
- Have a salad with non-starchy organic vegetables in the evening
- Avoid exercising
- Supplemental protein drinks can be consumed

## *Juice Cleanse Detox Diet*

This detox diet involves consuming only juices from fruits and vegetables as a means of detoxifying the body and losing weight. Juicing involves squeezing the juice from vegetables and fruits while separating them from the pulp. This is different from blending, which includes mixing all the edible parts of the vegetables and fruits, including the pulp. This detox method is controversial as it restricts several food groups and calories. However, many people swear by its benefits.

The rules for following this detox diet include:

- It must be done for a period ranging from 3 to 10 days
- The practitioner must drink only liquids and juices for the detox.
- Dietary supplements must be taken in combination to juicing.
- Juicing can be combined with other colon cleansing methods such as colonic irrigation or enemas

## **The Benefits of Practicing the Juice Clean Detox Diet**

- Obtaining high amounts of vitamins and minerals

- Boosted immune system
- Boosted energy
- Decreased risk of inflammation
- Improved digestion
- Lowered blood sugar levels
- Improved nutrient absorption
- Aids in lowering bad cholesterol levels
- Faster weight loss
- Helps boosts athletic performance

To help you gain these benefits, here is a list of fruits and vegetables that can be juiced in combinations to provide maximum efficiency in the detoxing process:

- Spinach. This has anti-cancer properties and is packed in vitamins. Its mild flavor can be disguised by adding other ingredients.
- Kale. Kale is a powerful antioxidant and anti-inflammatory agent. It also aids in relieving the symptoms of arthritis and autoimmune diseases.
- Cucumber. This vegetable is made of 95% water and has powerful functions in detoxifying the kidney and liver.
- Carrots. This aids in improving eye health and lowering cholesterol in addition to being a good source of fiber, potassium, Vitamin K, and beta carotene.
- Beets. This also helps fight inflammation and lowers blood pressure.
- Celery. This has a high water content and is a good source of fiber, Vitamin K, Vitamin C, and Vitamin A.
- Ginger. This aids in supporting a healthy immune

system and digestive system.

- Oranges. In addition to being high in Vitamin C and low in calories, this is an immune system booster.
- Apples. This aids in supporting cardiovascular health and is an anti-inflammatory agent.
- Lemon. This is a highly effective cleansing agent and cuts through the bitterness of using greens like kale.

## Juicing Recipes

Below you will find a list of ingredients for tasty and highly detoxifying recipes. Remember that all vegetables and fruits need to be washed thoroughly before use and cut into ½-inch chunks. All peels should be removed. A high-quality juicer should be used, and the veggies and fruits should be juiced according to the manufacturer's instructions. All of these recipes can be served at room temperature or chilled.

### Carrot Spinach Juice Recipe

- 4 small carrots
- 1 cup of spinach
- 1 cup of parsley
- ½ apple

This recipe is great for achieving clear skin.

### Green Juice Recipe

- 1 lemon
- 1 inch size piece fresh ginger
- 2 green apples
- 4 kale leaves
- 1 small cucumber

- 1 celery stalk

**Pink Grapefruit Juice Recipe**

- 1 pink grapefruit
- 2 oranges
- 1 head romaine lettuce
- 4 mint leaves

This detoxifying juice recipe promotes weight loss.

**The Ultimate Green Apple Detox Juice Recipe**

- 2 green apples
- 2 celery stalks with no leaves
- 1 small cucumber
- 6 kale leaves
- 1 inch piece fresh ginger
- ½ lemon

**Red Breakfast Juice Recipe**

- 2 beets
- 2 apples
- 2 carrots
- 2 lemons

## *Sugar Detox Diet*

This detox diet involves limiting the amount of sugar that is consumed daily. Practicing this diet is intended to purge the body of unhealthy sugar. This diet can be practiced for a few days, but the practitioner cannot simply revert to consuming sugars indiscriminately after a few days have passed. As a result, some people choose to permanently practice this diet.

## Types of Sugar

Sugar comes in different forms and they include:

### Fructose

This is the type of sugar that is naturally found in fruit. Even though consuming fruits is healthy, consuming too much fructose can have a negative impact on your health. This negative impact arises because fructose is broken down in the liver, which turns this into compounds such as triglycerides that can cause damage to the liver, free radicals that can damage body cells, and uric acid that can damage the arteries.

### Sucrose

This is the type of sugar commonly referred to as table sugar. It is the type of sugar that is added to baked goods, candy, and most other sugary foods that we consume. This sugar is a combination of fructose and another type of sugar called glucose. When the sugar is broken down into these two individual parts, glucose causes a spike in blood sugar levels.

### Glucose

This is the sugar molecule that the body commonly uses to derive energy. Glucose does not need to be consumed because the body naturally breaks down carbohydrates to form the molecule. Having too much glucose in the system causes an unhealthy rise in blood sugar levels.

### High fructose corn syrup

This is made from cornstarch and is composed of glucose and fructose just like sucrose.

## Why is a Sugar Detox Necessary?

This is not an easy diet to undergo, simply because sugar is an addictive substance. However, it is worth limiting its consumption because it has been linked to a number of medical conditions such as type 2 diabetes, heart disease, mental illness, and obesity.

Because sugar is such a highly addictive substance, people will experience withdrawal symptoms when practicing the sugar detox diet. Mental withdrawal symptoms include depression, anxiety, problems focusing and concentrating, changes in sleep pattern, and sugar cravings. Physical withdrawal symptoms include lightheadedness, dizziness, fatigue, nausea, and tingling of the skin.

To fight this withdrawal symptoms, here are a few tips you can employ:

- Quit sugar cold turkey
- Increase your fiber intake
- Eat more protein
- Avoid using artificial sweeteners
- Get rid of junk food and processed foods in your home
- Drink more water
- Exercise regularly
- Manage your stress levels
- Consumer green vegetables
- Get good quality and quantity sleep

**Health benefits of Decreased Sugar Consumption**

- Improved dental health
- Decreased risk of developing cardiovascular diseases
- Improved focus and concentration
- Lowered blood sugar; therefore, lower the risk of developing type 2 diabetes

- Weight loss
- Reduced inflammation
- Boosted energy
- More mindful eating

**How to Practice the Sugar Detox Diet**

Remember that the first few days of the sugar detox diet can be trying due to sugar withdrawal and its associated symptoms, but with some effort you can make it through to the healthier side. Here are a few tips you can employ to make your sugar detox diet a success:

- Consume at least 45 grams of protein when you eat breakfast. This will allow you to feel full throughout the day.
- Include protein in every meal that you eat. Healthy protein options include eggs, fish, and plant-based sources like beans and tofu.
- Limit the amount of red meat that you consume.
- Do not consume processed meats like bacon and cold cuts.
- Include green leafy vegetables in every meal.
- Include between 45 and 75 grams of healthy fats such as avocado, salmon, flaxseeds, olive, and olive oil every day.
- Limit the consumption of fruits.
- Avoid processed foods such as crackers and chips

# Additional Ways to Help Your Body Detox

After you have practice whatever detoxification method that

you chose, be sure to keep your body cleansed by following the practices mentioned below:

- Eat more foods with Vitamin C or take a supplement. This vitamin helps the body produce a compound in the liver that drives toxins away. This compound is called glutathione.
- Drink the recommended number of glasses of water every day. This allows the better transport of nutrients to the different parts of your body in addition to eliminating false hunger and hydrating your cells.
- Practice deep breathing technique to ensure that oxygen circulates completely throughout your body.
- Manage your stress levels by managing your work/home life, practicing meditation techniques like yoga, and being grateful every day.
- Eat a lot of fiber through plant-based sources, such as beets, radishes, broccoli and artichokes.
- Keep the liver cleansed by drinking green tea and consuming herbs like dandelion root and milk thistle.
- Sweat in the sauna so that your body can eliminate toxins through perspiration.
- Get plenty of exercise so that your body can detoxify itself through perspiration.
- Remove toxins through your pores by dry brushing your skin or trying detoxifying foot spas and baths.
- Practice hydrotherapy. This is the practice of taking a very warm shower for five minutes and allowing the water to run down your back. This is followed up by allowing cold water to wash over your body for 30 seconds. Repeat this three times then get into bed for 30

minutes.
- Limit alcohol intake.
- Limit caffeine intake. Drinking caffeinated drink brings your body to a more acidic state. Decreasing the intake allows the body to be more alkaline, which is more conducive to detoxing.

Be sure to consult your doctor before you start practicing any detox diet.

# Chapter 7:
# Plant-Based Diet

With the word "diet" being thrown around so easily these days, it can seem overwhelming when choosing the one that is right for you. With the many benefits that plants afford us medicinally, it only makes sense to try a plant-based diet to reap the benefits of such clean eating. However, before we delve into the topic of plant-based eating, let's take a look at processed foods and why they are bad for your health.

## What are Processed Foods?

A processed food is any food that has been altered in some way during the preparation process to make it more flavorful, convenient, or shelf-stable. There are various degrees of processing foods.

### *Types of Food Processing*

The NOVA classification system, which was introduced in 2009, lists food processing in four categories. They are:

- Unprocessed or minimally processed foods. These foods are still in their natural state by the end of the processing. Unprocessed foods are naturally edible parts of a plant or animal. Minimally processed foods are altered slightly. This is usually done to extend the shelf-life of the foods. For example, pre-cut green beans are processed foods; however, they look almost the same as you would find them in nature. Processes that alter minimally processed foods include cleaning, freezing,

- Processed culinary ingredients. These are food ingredients that are derived from minimally-processed foods through processes such as refining, pressing, and grinding. These ingredients are not usually eaten on their own by used to prepare other dishes. They include plant-based oils, flour, pasta made from whole grains, seeds, and nuts.
- Processed foods. There are foods that are from either of the first two categories to which fat, sugar, or salt has been added. There are usually ready to eat without preparation and contain at least two ingredients. Examples included canned fish, canned fruits, and some cheeses.
- Heavily processed foods. These are also called ultra-processed foods. They have been chemically altered with additives, artificial flavors, and other ingredients. They are prepared beyond the addition of fat, sugar, and salt. Examples include chips, cookies, and some frozen dinner and breakfast cereals. Highly-processed foods pose the highest danger to health because they were prepared with ingredients made to increase cravings and overeating.

## Properties of Highly-Processed Foods

- They are usually filled with sugar, which can go by other names such as high fructose corn syrup. While our bodies do use sugars to gain energy, most of these added sugars are empty calories that contain no real nutritional value. In addition, consuming too much sugar can lead to devastating health consequences, such as unhealthy weight gain and increased risk of developing cardiovascular diseases. Also, sugar is a highly addictive substance. In fact, sugar is almost ten times as addictive as cocaine. This is why we find it so hard to keep away from sugars and junk food in general.

- They are usually stripped of fiber. Fiber helps us feel full faster, which allows us to consume fewer calories. Fiber also helps with the absorption of carbohydrates. The lack of fiber in highly processed foods makes these foods go through the digestive system quicker, which makes it more difficult for the body to feel satisfied. This leads to the consumption of larger meals and more frequent meals, which leads to unhealthy weight gain in addition to other negative health consequences.

- They usually contain additives. An additive is a substance that is added to food to alter its taste, appearance, or shelf life. Unfortunately, these additives stimulate the reward system in the brain by activating the release of the neurotransmitter called dopamine. Dopamine is a feel-good hormone that makes the person attached to these processed foods. This attachment makes it harder to stop eating them.

- They typically contain several ingredients that are hard to pronounce. These ingredients are artificial and are used to enhance flavor, extended shelf-life or improve the texture of the product. The terms are even masked by generating names such as artificial flavor.

- They can contain high levels of sodium. Salt is added to highly-processed food to improve the taste and texture and increase shelf-life. While the body does need sodium to function at optimum capacity, too much salt can increase sodium levels in the blood to an unsafe level and elevate the risk of developing cardiovascular diseases and high blood pressure.

- Highly processed foods are typically extremely low in nutritional value compared to unprocessed or minimally processed foods. This is because the processing procedure strips these foods of their nutritional value. Even though synthetic minerals and vitamins are added to replace those lost during the process of manufacturing these goods, they cannot compare to the original nutrients.

- They often contain trans fats and processed oils. This is because they are often manufactured with refined seed and vegetable oils that are hydrogenated. This is done because it is a cheap alternative that increases the shelf-life of these foods. Trans fats are unhealthy to consume and can lead to inflammation and unhealthy weight gain.

## *The Health Risk Associated With Eating Heavily Processed Foods*

- Highly processed foods can alter moods. Most people have heard of the term hangry, which is an emotionally aggressive state that some people suffer from when they are hungry or deprived of a particular snack or food. This is because of the addictive nature of processed food, which increases irritability and aggression. In addition, consuming highly processed foods contributes to the development of mental illnesses such as anxiety and depression.

- Processed foods can disrupt the consumer's sleep patterns. Consuming too many sugars and salts make it hard to fall asleep and stay asleep. This is because of the energy spikes and crashes that are related to fluctuating blood sugar and insulin levels.

- Processed foods increase the risk of becoming obese. Because processed foods are easy to grab, addictive in nature and do not make us feel as full. this usually leads to overeating. This can lead to unhealthy weight gain, which can lead to obesity. Obesity is a disease that develops from having too much body fat. Obesity is different from being overweight, which can mean that a person simply weighs too much. Bones, fat, and retained water can contribute to a person being overweight. Obesity is not a disease that happens in isolation but occurs in conjunction with a host of other diseases such as diabetes, heart disease, and certain cancers.

- Consuming highly-processed food increases the risk of developing certain types of cancer.

- Eating highly-processed foods increases the risk of developing metabolic diseases, such as diabetes and irritable bowel syndrome.

## *How to Reduce the Amount of Processed Foods in Your Diet*

Because processed foods are available in such a high number and variety, it is difficult for the everyday man and woman to avoid them. However, there are a few practices that you can use to reduce the amount of processed foods that you consume on a daily basis. These practices include:

- Checking the labels of the foods that you purchase. Typically processed foods have a longer ingredients list compared to minimally or unprocessed foods. They also typically have ingredients that are hard to pronounce. Watch out for these, and try to stick to foods that have a short list of ingredients and ingredients that you can pronounce and are familiar with.

- Keep food shopping at grocery stores to a minimum. Whole food markets at a great area to locate minimally or unprocessed foods. Typically grocery stores stock tons of packaged foods that are highly processed.

- Try to avoid highly processed meats such as bacon and sausage, and choose minimally-processed meats such as seafood and chicken breast.

- Cook at home more often. This gives you more control of your diet compared to eating out at restaurants. To make this easier to do, you can cook in batches and keep your meals frozen so that you can dine on tasty leftovers any day of the week.

- Practice a food plant-based diet. Plant-based diets revolve around eating foods that are derived from plants while keeping processed foods to a minimum if they are not avoided altogether.

# What is a Plant-Based Diet?

A plant-based diet is one that emphasizes the consumption of whole vegetables and fruits and whole grains while minimizing the intake of processed foods and animal products. It is a common misconception that a plant-based diet is one that is either vegan or vegetarian. While there are many similarities between the three diets, they are not synonymous.

Those who follow the vegan diet abstain from consuming animal products, including eggs, honey, seafood and dairy. On the other hand, vegetarians exclude all meat and poultry from their diets but still consume some animal products, such as dairy, eggs and seafood. A plant-based diet, on the other hand, offers more flexibility. While practitioners consume mostly plant products, animal products are not completely off-limit, even though the practitioner may choose to exclude all animal products or consume only small amounts of meat, dairy, eggs, poultry, and seafood. The beauty of this diet is that it holds no strict guidelines. The only rule is that the practitioner focuses on eating fresh foods derived from plant sources and minimizing processed and animal-based foods.

## What Can be Eaten on the Plant-Based Diet

Since the plant-based diet is so flexible, many people find that they can eat a lot of foods that they enjoyed before. Even if it is dramatically different, such as in cases where the person consumed mostly processed foods, then I have made locating the things that you can and cannot eat a cinch. This list can double as a shopping list.

## Plant-Based Shopping List

### Fruits

These include pears, mangoes, bananas, pineapple, oranges, limes, lemons, tangerines, berries, peaches, grapes, plums, watermelon, jackfruit, cantaloupe, avocados, apples, cherries, honeydew, and kiwi.

### Dried fruits

Dried fruits include raspberries, raisins, prunes, dates, apricots, and mango.

### Vegetables

Vegetables include cauliflower, broccoli, squash, eggplant, zucchini, tomatoes, spinach, kale, carrots, asparagus, peppers, sweet potatoes, potatoes, eggplant, celery, radish, onions, mushrooms, cucumber, cabbage, Brussel sprouts, artichoke hearts, turnips, lettuce, collard greens, arugula, bok choy, beets, yams, pumpkins, corn, and parsnip.

**Whole grains**

These include rolled oats, quinoa, brown rice, whole grain pasta, barley, farro, couscous, cornmeal, rye, buckwheat, millet, spelt, bulgur, and whole grain tortillas.

**Seeds and nuts**

These include almonds, cashews, macadamia, pumpkin seeds, sunflower seeds, Brazil nuts, Hazelnuts, Flaxseeds, pine nuts, sesame seeds, pecans, hemp seeds, chia seeds, walnuts, and teff.

**Nut butters**

Nut butters include tahini, cashew butter, peanut butter, macadamia butter, pistachio butter, hazelnut butter, almond butter, walnut butter, and pecan butter.

**Plant-based milks**

These include coconut milk, almond milk, cashew milk, and soymilk.

**Plant-based proteins**

These include tofu, edamame, and tempeh.

**Healthy fats**

Healthy fats include olive oil, coconut oil, avocado oil, unsweetened coconut, grapeseed oil, rice bran oil, coconut butter, canola oil, and macadamia oil.

**Legumes and beans**

These include chickpeas, lentils, peanuts, black beans, black-eye peas, kidney beans, lima beans, whites beans, pinto beans, mung beans, and garbanzos.

**Sweeteners**

Sweeteners include beet sugar, dates, coconut sugar, agave nectar, brown rice syrup, maple syrup, stevia, raw cane sugar, palm sugar, and sylitol.

**Unsweetened beverages**

Beverages include tea, coffee, water, and sparkling water.

**Herbs and spices**

These include black pepper, salt, basil, rosemary, curry, turmeric, cumin, cilantro, chives, dill, garlic, green onion, ginger, nutmeg, cinnamon, chili powder, thyme, parsley, paprika, and oregano.

**Miscellaneous items**

These include capers, olives, mustard, balsamic vinegar, apple cider vinegar, white wine vinegar, rice vinegar, white vinegar, seaweed, miso paste, sauerkraut, nutritional yeast, kimchi, amino acids, red wine vinegar, baking soda, baking powder, and cornstarch.

If you choose to add a few animal-based products to your diet, here are a few guidelines:

- Poultry: choose free-range, organic sources.
- Dairy and eggs: use organic products obtained from animals raised in pastures.
- Seafood: obtain wild-caught sources from sustainable fisheries.
- Pork and beef: obtain grass-fed or pasture-raised sources.

## Foods to Use in Small Quantities

- Eggs
- Dairy

- Beef
- Pork
- Chicken
- Seafood
- Lamb
- Game meats

**Foods to Avoid**

- Processed foods like packaged foods (crackers, frozen dinners, chips, and cereal bars)
- Foods with added sugars like soda, candy, cereal with high sugar content, and cookies.
- Refined grains like white bread, white rice, and refined pasta.
- Fast foods like hot dogs, chicken nuggets, cheeseburgers, and fried chicken.
- Processed animal products like sausage, beef jerky, lunch meat, and bacon.
- Artificial sweeteners like Splenda and Equal.

# Benefits to Practicing a Plant-Based Diet

There are several health benefits to practicing a plant-based diet, and they include:

- Lowering the risk of unhealthy weight gain and overeating. People who practice a plant-based diet tend to feel full faster; therefore, they eat smaller portions. In addition, the calories they consume are burned quickly and cleanly. When practiced with an exercise regimen, a plant-based diet can help slim you down easily and without fuss.

- Lowering the risk of developing cardiovascular diseases, such as heart disease and stroke. Consuming fruits, vegetables, whole grains, nuts, seeds, and legumes provide the body with good cholesterol while lowering the levels of bad cholesterol, which is a major contributing factor to the development of poor cardiovascular health.

- Aids in decreasing inflammation within the body. Consuming raw plant-based foods that are rich in antioxidants and probiotics helps to decrease the symptoms of rheumatoid arthritis, which includes swelling, morning stiffness, and joint pain.

- Offers protection against certain types of cancer such as breast, colon, and prostate cancer. Consuming legumes on a regular basis, consuming soy-based products, and eliminating or minimizing the consumption of animal products helps in the risk reduction of developing these cancers.

- Allows the practitioner to consume high amounts of nutrients such as fiber, antioxidants, vitamins such as Vitamin C, Vitamin D, Vitamin K, Vitamin D and vitamin E, and minerals such as magnesium, folate, and potassium.

# How to Transition to a Plant-Based Diet

Starting a new diet can be hard and requires some planning, effort, and maybe even willpower. There are a few strategies that you can employ to make your transition to a plant-based diet easier:

- Know what your motivation for practicing a plant-based diet is. It may be that you want to eat healthier. It may also be that you want to leave a smaller environmental footprint as this is one of the benefits of practicing a plant-based diet. It may be because you want to enhance the medicinal benefits you gain from using herbal medicine. Whatever your motivation is, write it down and remind yourself regularly of why you have changed your diet.

- Stop slowly by picking a few plant-based meals and rotating them throughout the week. Oatmeal, stir-fried veggies, beans, and brown rice bowls and lentil soup are a great starting point. Another great option for starting slow is to switch up only one meal for the week, such as breakfast, to a plant-based option.

- Eat variety. Practicing a plant-based diet does not mean that you eat only carrots every day. With the thousands of options in fruit, veggies and whole grains available, you can switch it up every day so that your palette get something rewarding, and you do not get bored.

- Rid your kitchen cabinets of processed foods. It is easy to reach for something that is in easy reach, so cleaning out your cupboards of processed food makes it easier to transition to a plant-based diet. Instead, stock up your shelves and refrigerator with healthy, unprocessed, or minimally-processed foods.

- Ensuring that you have plant-based options to get in your daily recommended value of protein. By minimizing or avoiding proteins obtained from animal sources such as meat and eggs, you may come up with a deficit of protein in your diet. But you can quickly fill up this gap with plant-based protein options, such as chickpeas, nuts, seeds, legumes, tofu and tempeh.

- Keep on educating yourself about plant-based eating. Even in this age of technology, it is easy to become misinformed due to false information being published at the click of a finger. It is important that you keep yourself informed from reliable sources so that you can properly plan your plant-based diet.

- Surround yourself with like-minded people. Humans are social creatures and tend to be impacted by the crowd that they run with. It is easy to feel isolated if you are the only one practicing a plant-based diet in a crowd that consumes processed foods regularly. Therefore, to ensure that you do not yield to social pressure to revert to a diet of processed foods, it is a great idea to find like-minded people who practice a plant-based diet and medicine. You do not even need to leave your house to do this as social media has made it easy to find people with similar interests.
- Plan your meals. Having weekly meal plans are great for keeping you on track with your eating since they take the guesswork out of what you will eat daily. To help get you started, please find the sample 7-day meal plan below.

# 7-Day Plant-Based Meal Plan

## Day 1

Breakfast: Chickpea omelette

Lunch: Chickpea salad topped with fresh chopped veggies, avocado, and pumpkin seeds

Dinner: Zucchini curry

Snack 1: Kale chips

Snack 2: Carrot sticks dipped in roasted tahini veggie dip

## Day 2

Breakfast: Coconut milk oatmeal topped with coconut flakes, berries, and walnuts

Lunch: No-meat butternut squash chili

Dinner: Cauliflower rice stir-fry

Snack 1: Coconut chips

Snack 2: Parmesan popcorn

## Day 3

Breakfast: Chocolate banana pancakes

Lunch: Quinoa topped with veggies and feta

Dinner: Black bean and sweet potato tacos

Snack 1: Sweet potato chips

Snack 2: Celery sticks dipped in cashew butter

## Day 4

Breakfast: Almond banana granola served with coconut milk

Lunch: Hummus veggie wraps

Dinner: Gluten-free vegan macaroni and cheese

Snack 1: Tofu chips

Snack 2: Granola

## Day 5

Breakfast: Overnight oats topped with chia seeds and fresh berries

Lunch: Vegan BLT sandwich

Dinner: Grilled tempeh with roasted broccoli and potatoes

Snack 1: Trail mix

Snack 2: Fresh fruit like banana or pear slices

## *Day 6*

Breakfast: Blueberry muffins

Lunch: Cauliflower and lentil curry

Dinner: Eggplant lasagna with green salad

Snack 1: Roasted chickpeas

Snack 2: Berry banana smoothie

## *Day 7*

Breakfast: Kale blackberry smoothie with cashew butter and coconut milk

Lunch: Tahini quinoa and roasted veggies

Dinner: Black bean burgers

Snack 1: Dried figs

Snack 2: Apple slices dipped in peanut butter

# Chapter 8:
# Essentials Oils

It is common to hear essential oils and aromatherapy used in conjunction with each other, but many people do not understand the tremendous positive impact that both can have on their lives. This chapter is dedicated to explaining what are essential oils and their health benefits in addition to giving you a comprehensive list of the different types and the effects. It should be noted that essential oils do not work for everyone, yet some people swear by the medicinal effects it afforded them. There is no harm in trying them to see if they work for you.

## What are Essential Oils?

Essential oils are the resulting ingredient when compounds have been extracted from plants. They are so called because they capture the 'essence' or scent of the plant. Essential oils are created through the process of distillation, which uses steam or water or a mechanical methods like cold-pressing. Once the aromatic compounds have been extracted from the plant, they are combined with a carrier oil to create a final product.

A carrier oil is also created from a plant; however, it is used to dilute essential oils so that they can be carried on your skin. Essential oils are very potent and can cause irritation if they are applied directly to the skin. Examples of carrier oils include olive oil, black seed oil, avocado oil, sunflower oil, sweet almond oil, grapeseed oil, and coconut oil. They are unscented or lightly scented and do not interfere with the function of the essential oil. They are nourishing to skin. Essential oils are used by inhaling or applying topically to skin. They should never be swallowed.

# The History of Essential Oil Use

Essential oils and aromatherapy originated in Ancient Egypt. Egyptians cultivated plants to create oils that were used in cosmetic, medicinal, and religious purposes. These oils were also used for embalming.

These oils were extracted through a solvent extraction method using animal fat in the early stage of the use of essential oils. However, there is evidence that the distillation process has been used since 3500 BC.

It was not long after, Indian and Chinese cultures started exploring the use of aromatherapy. The practices of the Egyptians were adopted by the Greeks around 400 BC. It was introduced by well-known physician Hippocrates, who was a firm believer of using holistic practices to treat patients. This knowledge was then adopted by the Romans to promote good health. Aromatic baths were especially popular at that time.

The use of essential oils went through a dark period after the fall of the Roman Empire. It was repressed by religious denominations that considered bathing a sin. The use of aromatics to cover stench was practiced, and the practices that Hippocrates encouraged were forgotten.

Luckily, there was a rebirth of interest in aromatherapy and essential oil usage in the Renaissance period. A physician called Paracelsus (1493-1541) helped with this introduction by claiming to "cure leprosy" with the use of plant extracts. The term aromatherapy was then invented by a French chemist and perfumer called Rene Maurice Gattefosse in 1937.

Interest in aromatherapy exploded in the late 70s and early 80s due to a boom in interest in natural medicine.

# What is Aromatherapy?

Aromatherapy is also called essential oil therapy. It is a holistic approach to promoting good health and wellness through the use of natural plant extracts. These essential oils improve health mentally, physically, and emotionally through the medicinal properties of these oils. Essential oil therapy has been used by humans for thousands of years and was popular in ancient cultures, such as Egyptian, Indian and Chinese. Its benefits can still be gained today.

## *Benefits of Aromatherapy and Essential Oils*

- Helps improve digestion
- Aids in pain management
- Improves sleep quality and helps fight insomnia
- Soothes sore joints
- Treats migraines and headaches
- Aids in easing the discomfort of child labor
- Helps alleviate the side effects of chemotherapy
- Reduces inflammation
- Reduces stress and anxiety
- Aids in the treatment of asthma
- Helps reduce PMS and menopausal symptoms
- Aids in reducing the symptoms of arthritis
- Aids in treating erectile dysfunction
- Can be used an antibiotic and antimicrobial agent

Aromatherapy affords these benefits through the smell of and the skin absorption of the essential oils. Aromatherapy works by using the following products, which can be used in combination or alone:

- Inhalers
- Diffusers
- Aroma spritzers
- Body oils, lotions, and creams
- Facial steamers
- Clay masks
- Hot and cold compresses
- Bath salts

# How Essential Oils Work

When essential oils are inhaled, they stimulate specific areas in the limbic system. The limbic system is a part of the brain where emotions, long-term memory, sense of smell, and behavior are controlled. It is interesting that this part of the brain aids in forming memories and regulating emotions as it explains why certain smells trigger memories or emotions in some people.

The limbic system also helps to control some unconscious bodily functions, such as heart rate, blood pressure and breathing. The use of essential oils has been reported to enhance or help regulate some of these functions by some users.

When essential oils are applied to the skin, they are absorbed to interact with the body in a variety of ways.

# Other Uses of Essential Oils

In addition to be used in aromatherapy, essential oils have the following uses:

- To freshen up the scent of homes, cars, and offices
- To freshen up the scent of laundry
- As an insect repellent
- To add a natural scent to homemade cosmetics
- To extend the shelf-life of some foods

# Types of Essential Oils and the Part of the Plant That They Are Derived From

Essential oils can be derived from one part of a plant or several parts of the plant.

### *Derived from the leaves*

- Bay laurel
- Bergamot mint
- Cajeput
- Cinnamon
- Eucalyptus
- Geranium
- Lemon Myrtle
- Myrtle
- Niaouli
- Ravensara
- Tea tree
- Tobacco

- Violet

***Derived from the flowers***

- Boronia
- Chamomile
- Clove
- Diwana
- Jasmine
- Lindale blossom
- Rose
- Tuberose
- Ylang ylang

***Derived from flowering herbs***

The oils are created through the distillation of both the flowers and the leaves. They include:

- Basil
- Catnip
- Holy basil
- Hyssop
- Lavender
- Lavandin
- Lemon balm
- Marjoram
- Oregano
- Peppermint
- Rosemary

- Sage
- Spearmint
- Thyme
- Yarrow

**Derived from the bark**

- Cassia
- Cinnamon

**Derived from the wood**

- Amyris
- Cedarwood
- Palo Santo
- Rosewood
- Sandalwood

**Derived from the needles**

- Cypress
- Fir
- Scotch pine
- Spruce

**Derived from the grass**

- Citronella
- Lemongrass
- Palmarosa

**Derived from citrus rinds**

- Bergamot

- Grapefruit
- Lemon
- Lime
- Mandarin
- Orange
- Tangerine

**Derived from the gum, resin, or balsam**

- Benzoin
- Peru balsam
- Elemi
- Galbanum
- Gurjum

**Derived from berries or fruit**

- Allspice
- Black pepper
- Juniper berry
- May Chang

**Derived from moss or lichen**

- Oak moss

**Derived from Roots**

- Angelica
- Ginger
- Vetiver

### *Derived from seeds*

- Ambrette
- Anise
- Cardamom
- Carrot
- Coffee bean
- Coriander
- Cumin
- Dill
- Fennel
- Nutmeg
- Parsley

# Popular Essential Oils and Their Health Benefits

- Angelica root. This helps support a healthy immune and respiratory system in addition to fighting stress, fatigue, and tension. It also aids in restoring strength and stamina.
- Bergamot. This helps reduce stress and improve certain skin conditions like eczema.
- Black pepper. The spicy scent aids in soothing muscle aches, supports a healthy digestive system, and stimulates appetite.
- Cajeput. This aids in treating skin conditions like insect bites, blemishes, and excess oil production. It also aids in relieving minor joint and muscle pain.

- Chamomile. Best essential oil aids in improving mood and promoting relaxation.
- Citronella. This is a mosquito repellent.
- Eucalyptus. This essential oil aids in clearing congestion and is an anti-inflammatory.
- Geranium. This helps relieve hormonal headaches.
- Jasmine. This is in alleviating the pains of childbirth, enhances libido, and fights depression.
- Lavender. It aids in relieving stress and helps soothe allergy-related symptoms. It is also an anti-inflammatory agent and helps relieve migraines.
- Lemon. Lemon oil helps improve mood, treats headaches, and improve digestion.
- Peppermint. Aids in digestion and boosts energy. It is also an anti-inflammatory and helps relieve tension headaches.
- Rose. This is essential oil is in reducing anxiety and improving mood.
- Sandalwood. This essential oil is improving focus and concentration in addition to calming nerves. It also helps relieve the symptoms of allergies, such as runny nose and sneezing.
- Ylang ylang. This is in the treatment of certain skin conditions, nausea, and headaches.

# The Dangers of Improper Usage of Essential oils

The benefits that essential oils can afford are numerous and far-reaching. However, if essential oils are used incorrectly, they can cause poisoning even if small amounts are ingested.

Essential oils are not fit for consumption and should always be diluted with carrier oils to decrease the potency. If this is not done, allergic reactions, skin rashes and burns are possible. Children are especially susceptible. The severity of the toxicity that an essential oil has depends on the type of oil and the amount that has been ingested. Symptoms of toxicity include:

- Seizures
- Persistent coughing
- Nausea
- Vomiting
- Diarrhea
- Skin irritation
- Redness, irritation, or pain in the eyes
- Drowsiness
- Shallow breathing
- Coma in cases where a large amount has been ingested

Luckily, there are steps you can take to minimize the damage in case of exposure. If the essential oil has been swallowed, rinse out the mouth and call your local poison information center. Do not intake any oral fluids until that is advised by the local poison information center. Ingesting fluids can cause aspiration of fluid into the lungs or vomiting, which should not be induced.

If eye exposure to essential oil occurs, immediately rinse out the eyes using running water. Allow the flowing water to run from the corner of the eye closest to the nose over the eye and outward. They should be done for 15 minutes, and the eye should be evaluated by a licensed medical doctor.

If excessive inhalation of essential oil occurs, the affected person should be taken into an open area where they can breathe in fresh air. If this does not help in settling the symptoms, the local poison information center should be called.

If pure essential oil is exposed to the skin, then the skin should be washed with clean water and soap after all contaminated clothing has been removed. If the symptoms are not resolved by this, a licensed medical doctor should be seen.

Essential oils should be handled with caution and only after they have been properly diluted with carrier oils. Extra caution should be taken when essential oils are handled by pregnant and breastfeeding women and children.

# The Do's and Don'ts of Using Essential Oil Safely

### The Do's

When purchasing essential oils, check the quality to ensure that any extra ingredients added are not detrimental to your health. Not all added ingredients are bad, so you simply need to be vigilant.

Test a small bit of the essential oil on a small part of your arm or leg before using large amounts. This will allow you to see how you skin responds. Some people have had skin irritation and an allergic reaction to using essential oils.

Stop the use of essential oil immediately if you notice undesirable skin reactions, such as rashes, itchiness, and little bumps. This applies even if the essential oil is an ingredient in another produce like a cream. Wash the product off with soap and clean water.

Store essential oils correctly. They should be kept at room temperature in a dry area that is out of reach of young children.

## *The Don'ts*

Do not rub essential oils on your body indiscriminately. They are not safe to put in your nose, eyes, mouth, or private areas. The arms and legs are safe application areas.

Do not apply essential oils to damaged skin. This doubly applies to undiluted essential oils. The application of essential oils to inflamed or injured skin can cause adverse skin reactions.

Do not keep or use essential oils that are more than three years old. Past this point the essential oil would have likely spoiled due to oxygen exposure. Not only do the essential oils do not work as well, but they can cause allergies reaction or skin irritation. If you notice that your essential oil had changed in color, texture or smell, throw it out and replace it.

Do not overuse essential oil. The old adage that too much of a good thing is bad. Even when essential oils are diluted, they can cause a negative reaction when used too often or in amounts that are too large.

# Chapter 9: Herbal Medicine

## What are Medicinal Plants?

These are also referred to as medicinal herbs and have been used for illness prevention and cure since historic times. These are handy plants to keep around to treat common ailments, such as tummy aches, headaches, and even the symptoms of bug bites. They can be used in teas, as food garnishes, inhalants, and applied topically. This chapter is dedicated to providing you with a long list of medicinal plants that are great to keep around your home to keep your body in tip-top shape the natural way.

### *Common Medicinal Plants and their Health Benefits*

**Thyme**

Thyme is popular for use in cooking, but not many people know about its medicinal functions. Thyme health benefits include:

- Treating respiratory issues
- Supporting a healthy immune system
- Improving blood circulation
- Soothing sore throats and coughs

These benefits are made possible because of the presence of the compound called thymol in the plant. This compound has antifungal and antibacterial properties. These properties help in preventing foodborne diseases by decontaminating food and preventing infections from occurring in the body. Due to these properties, thymol is a common ingredient in vapor rubs and mouthwash. To benefit from thyme, you can brew its leaves for tea, use as a garnish for meals, or apply topically as a cream.

## Kava Kava

Kava kava goes by the scientific name of Piper methysticum. The name kava means bitter. The plant has been used by Pacific Islanders for thousands of years to:

- Reduce pain
- Reduce the risk of cancer
- Protect neurons from damage
- Reduce anxiety
- As a sleep aid

Kava kava is most often brewed as a tea.

## Echinacea

This is an herbaceous flowering plant from the daisy family that is found in Eastern and Central North America. It mainly grows in prairies and open wooded areas. This plant activates a chemical in the body that helps fight the symptoms of the cold and flu by decreasing inflammation in the body. In addition to fighting the common, echinacea also:

- Increases athletic performance
- Fights gingivitis
- Decreases anxiety
- Prevents the formation of anal warts that are caused by the human papilloma virus (HPV)
- Aids in treating indigestion
- Aids in treating yeast
- Acts as a pain reliever

- Fights migraine headaches
- Fights indigestion

## Sage

The official name of this plant is salvia officinalis. Sage is well known in the diabetic community for its ability to naturally lowering glucose levels. It also helps support memory and combats degenerative diseases. Sage can be used to prepare dishes as well as in beauty products. It's health benefits include:

- Supporting digestive health
- Strengthening the immune system
- Aiding in the treatment and management of diabetes
- Improving skin health
- Improving memory
- Enhancing overall brain function
- Supplying antioxidants

You can reap these benefits by brewing the fresh leaves for tea, inhaling it as an essential oil, applying the essential oil topically, and using as a garnish for meals.

## Rosemary

The official name of this medicinal plant is Rosmarinus officinalis. Rosemary is filled with essential vitamins and minerals that help to support the function of a healthy body in addition to medicinal benefits. Its medicinal benefits include:

- Supporting a healthy liver
- Support health hair growth
- Reducing inflammation
- Treating halitosis

- Improving memory
- Enhancing overall brain function
- Improving blood circulation

Gain these benefits by brewing the dried leaves for tea, applying the essential oil topically and using as a garnish for meals.

**Parsley**

Parsley, also known as petroselinum crispum, is known as a delicious garnish in the cooking world, but did you know that it helps support several of the body's essential systems such as the immune system? Because of it's high concentration of Vitamin K and antioxidants, it also aids in boosting overall body health. Parsley's health benefits include:

- Fighting halitosis
- Supporting bone health
- Relieving bloating
- Supporting digestive health
- Supplying antioxidants

In addition to using this as a garnish in dishes, it can be used to brew tea and create juices.

**Peppermint**

This herb is commonly found in toothpaste, gum and even in deserts, but its health benefits are numerous. They include:

- Treating halitosis
- Supporting digestive health
- As an antibacterial agent
- Relieving digestive issues such as gas indigestion and nausea

- Relieving headaches
- Soothing muscle pain
- Relieving allergies

These benefits can be obtained by brewing the leaves in tea, inhaling the essential oil, and applying the essential oil topically.

## Basil

The scientific name of Basil is ocimum basilicum. It is commonly used to add flavor to the dishes and as a garnish. Basil is rich in vitamins and minerals such as vitamin k and iron. This rich nutritional value helps combat common ailments. Basil's many health benefits include:

- Aiding in the metabolism of different compounds in the body
- Acting as an antibacterial agent
- Supplying the body with antioxidants
- Boosting immunity
- Improving digestion
- Strengthening bone and liver health
- Reducing inflammation
- Slowing the aging process
- Reducing stress

In addition to using basil as a garnish, it can be used as an ingredient to create smoothies.

## Catnip

The scientific name for catnip is nepeta cataria. Most people are familiar with catnip's role in attracting cats to roll around in it. This is because it is a stimulant for the animals. It also acts as a sedative if the cat consumes it. It has a variety of effects on humans, including being a sleep aid and a stress reliever. These effects come from the presence of compounds such as thymol and nepetalactone. The health benefits of catnip include:

- Reducing anxiety and stress
- Inducing calmness
- Accelerating the recovery from fevers and colds
- Relieving stomach aches
- Acting as a bug repellent
- Relieving skin irritation from bug bites

People can reap the benefits of catnip by brewing its leaves in tea, drying the leaves and burning to release the aroma and applying the leaves or essential oil topically.

**Chamomile**

Scientifically referred to as matricaria chamomilla, chamomile is great at relieving a variety of illnesses and elements because of his high concentration of antioxidants. Many people are familiar with chamomile as tea and use it to relax just before bed. Its other health benefits include:

- Relieving pain
- Reducing inflammation
- Relieving congestion
- Improving skin health
- Acting as a sleep aid

Chamomile can be used by brewing the dry leaves, inhaling as an essential oil, and applying topically.

## Cayenne Pepper

Best known for adding a spicy kick to a meal or drink, cayenne pepper goes by the scientific name of capsicum annuum. The main compound responsible for cayenne pepper's role as a medicinal plant is called capsaicin. It is responsible for the spicy nature of cayenne pepper but also the health benefits that include:

- Relieving pain
- Lowering cholesterol
- Improving blood circulation
- Easing upset stomach
- Aiding in digestion
- Boosting metabolism
- Detoxifying the body

While cayenne pepper can be consumed as a pill, it is commonly added to dressings, spice mixes, sauces, and other dishes.

## Dandelion

This plant goes by the scientific name of taraxacum. While it is known as a pesky weed, you may want to think twice before you pluck it out of your front yard. Many people do not know this, but the dandelion is edible and full of health benefits because of its high nutritional value that includes Vitamin C, Vitamin K, calcium, iron, and more. Even the dandelion root affords a person many great health benefits, which include:

- Improving skin health
- Treating skin infections
- Supporting bone health

- Treating and preventing urinary tract infections
- Detoxifying the liver
- Supporting liver health

Dandelion roots can be brewed as a tea and its leaves can be used as a garnish for dishes.

## Garlic

Garlic goes by the scientific name of allium sativum and is considered a super-plant for fighting infections and aiding in the improvement of overall health. The health benefits of garlic include:

- Lowering cholesterol and blood pressure
- Aiding preventing the development of degenerative diseases such as Alzheimer's and dementia
- Improve in digestive health
- Preventing the development of cardiovascular diseases such as heart disease
- Boosting the function of the immune system

Garlic can be consumed raw, cooked as an ingredient in dishes and used to garnish dishes.

## Marigold

Going by the scientific name of tagetes, this medicine of plant is known for its fragrant nature. It is chock-full of antioxidants and other health-boosts in compounds that make it a great choice to keep around your home. Its benefits include:

- Treating skin diseases
- Soothing skin infections
- Boosting eye health
- As an antibacterial and antiseptic agent

- Reducing inflammation
- Treating eye pain and infection

A person can gain these health benefits from marigold by brewing the dried flowers for tea, using as a garnish in dishes, or applying the essential oil or cream topically.

**Lemon Balm**

Known scientifically as Melissa officinalis, this must be Santa plant is delicious and contains a variety of compounds that aid in:

- Reducing anxiety and stress
- Soothing menstrual cramps
- Reducing inflammation
- Treating cold sores
- Soothing restless children

To gain these health benefits you know how lemon balm's leaves can be brewed as a tea, applied topically as an essential oil, or used to garnish dishes and desserts.

**Tulsi**

This is an aromatic perennial plant that goes by the scientific name of ocimum tenuiflorum. This plant is also called holy basil and is celebrated for its remarkable holistic healing properties. These remedies include:

- Providing protection against insect bites and bacteria
- Providing relief from colds, bronchitis, coughs, and fever
- Relief against indigestion
- Aids in curing malaria
- Headache relief

This plant can be brewed as a tea and used to make an essential oil. It is commonly used in ayurveda medicine and comes in four varieties. This plant is native to India and is widespread across the Southeast Asian tropics.

## Aloe vera

Aloe vera is a plant that is grown in tropical climates all around the world and is native to North America, Southern Europe, and the Canary islands. There are even records of its medicinal use dating back to ancient Egypt. This plant has a variety of medicinal uses including:

- Providing relief against sunburn
- Healing wounds
- Relieving heartburn
- Reducing inflammation
- Help slow the spread of breast cancer
- Can be used to maintain oral health
- Aids lowering blood sugar levels
- Works as a natural laxative
- Used to grow fuller, longer hair
- Helps fight acne breakouts

Aloe vera has over 500 species. The succulent plant is stemless.

## Ashwagandha

Translated in skerritt, ashwagandha means "smell of a horse." This meaning references the plants unique smell and its ability to increase body strength. The scientific name is withania somnifera, but it also goes by other names, including winter cherry and the Indian ginseng. The proven health benefits of this plant include:

- Fighting inflammation
- Fighting tumor growth
- Lowering blood sugar levels
- Lowering cortisol levels. Cortisol is a stress hormone that is released from the adrenal glands in response to stress and when blood sugar levels are too low. The release of cortisol can become a chronic problem if it is uncontrolled and has detrimental health effects.
- Aids in reducing anxiety and stress
- Helps boost testosterone levels
- Aids an increasing fertility in men
- Aids in increasing muscle mass and body strength

**Stevia**

In addition to being a natural sweetener, stevia has a host of medical uses. They include:

- Fighting cavities other oral problems
- Helping to control blood sugar levels
- Aids in fighting type 2 diabetes
- Helping to control weight gain
- Helping to lower blood pressure
- Helping to strengthen bones
- Aids in preventing upper respiratory infections.

Stevia is a perennial shrub that belongs to the sunflower family. It is indigenous to South America and has over 200 species. The compounds that gives stevia leaf its sweet taste are called stevioside and rebaudioside A. These compounds were isolated in 1931, but it was during World War II that stevia was promoted as an alternative to sugar when sugar was in short supply. Stevia was used by Japanese in the 1970s to replace the banned artificial sweetener called saccharine.

**Marsh mellow**

As the name suggests this is the plant from which marshmallows were once made from. However, apart from its use in the confectionery treat, the roots and leaves of this plant we used to treat aching muscles, bruises, insect bites, gastritis, inflammation of the urinary and respiratory mucous membranes, as a counter to excessive stomach acid production, and to treat bruises and sprains. The leaves of this plant are edible and can be fried, boiled, or added to salads.

# Probiotics

Probiotics are live yeast and bacteria that reside in your body and are good for you. They are especially prominent in your digestive system. Typically, when people think of bacteria, they think of disease and infection, but the body is filled with bacteria that aid in upkeeping health because they help keep your gut healthy. While the body does indeed contains bad bacteria, good gut health depends on keeping a balance of the good and bad bacteria.

## *Types of Probiotics*

- Lactobacillus. This is the type of probiotic that comes to mind when most people think of probiotic. It is commonly found in fermented foods and yogurt and can help people who are lactose intolerant. Different strains of lactobacillus can help stop diarrhea.

- Bifidobacterium. This type of probiotic is typically found in dairy products and can be used to ease the symptoms of irritable bowel syndrome (IBS) among several other conditions.

- Saccharomyces boulardii. This is a yeast. It helps fight diarrhea and other digestive issues.

## *Benefits of Probiotics*

Eating a variety of probiotic rich foods gains a person the following benefits:

- Reduced risk of developing cancer. Scientific research has shown that the disturbance of the balance between good bacteria and bad bacteria in the gut can cause the uncontrolled development of cells, which can lead to cancer. Promoting the balance of bacteria in the gut reduces this risk.

- Reduced the risk of developing inflammatory bowel disease (IBD). This too is a condition that depends on the balance of good and bad bacteria in the gut. Keeping the balance tipped on the side of probiotics aids in lowering the risk of developing the condition.

- Improved digestion. Probiotics speed up the digestion process by breaking down food faster so that it does not linger in the digestive system. The aid that probiotics provide reduces the risk of developing symptoms of Crohn's disease, irritable bowel syndrome (IBS), and constipation.

- Aid in diabetes management. Probiotics improve glycemic control and lipid metabolism in persons with type 2 diabetes.

- Reduced risk of developing metabolic diseases. Metabolic diseases include type 2 diabetes, liver disease, and obesity. The regular consumption of probiotics can prevent and aid in the management of these conditions.

- The maintenance of vaginal health. The vagina contains several bacteria and spermicides and contraceptives, and antibiotics can throw off the delicate balance that ensures good health of the tract. This can cause infection. Regular consumption of probiotics can restore the balance and prevent infections and other issues.

- Help in maintaining mental health. The health of your gut can influence your mental health. Therefore, a regular consumption of probiotics can reduce the symptoms of mental disorders such as anxiety and depression.
- Reduces side effects from antibiotics. More than 30% of people who take antibiotics develop the side effect of antibiotic-associated diarrhea. Taking probiotics alongside antibiotics can prevent the development of the side effects.

## *Plant-Based Probiotics*

While yogurt is one of the most popular sources of probiotics, there are plant-based options available. See below for just a few of these.

### Sauerkraut

This is simply fermented cabbage. It is created by finely cutting up cabbage and fermenting it in brine, which is a concentrate of salt water. It is rich in vitamin C, vitamin K and potassium, in addition to the probiotic, lactobacillus.

### Kimchi

This is also another fermented cabbage dish and only differs from sauerkraut through the addition of spices and a few vegetables. It is rich in vitamins, antioxidants, and the same type of probiotic as sauerkraut.

## Miso

This is a Japanese seasoning made from soybeans, fermented salt, and a fungus called koji. In addition to its probiotic health benefits, it helps lower the risk of developing breast cancer and having a stroke. It is rich in various nutritional components such as protein, fiber, vitamins, and minerals.

## Tempeh

This is a fermented soybean product that originated in Indonesia but is popular worldwide as a high-protein meat substitute. It is greatly used in vegan and vegetarian cooking.

## Pickles

Pickles are a vegetable that have been fermented in a brine solution. This fermenting process creates a probiotic-rich food. Almost any vegetable can be pickled, but some popular options include carrots, cucumbers, green beans, red bell peppers and cauliflower. These should be enjoyed in moderation because of their high sodium content, which can cause high blood pressure and water retention. To add extra flavor to pickles, herbs and spices, such as garlic, bay leaf, and coriander seeds can be added.

# List of Herbal Remedies

Below you will find a comprehensive list listed from A to Z of remedies and medicines that can prevent and treat everyday maladies and more serious conditions such as arthritis.

- Alfalfa. This can be used to lower cholesterol, in addition to treating kidney and urinary tract ailments.
- Aloe vera. This can be used to treat skin infections and heal burns and wounds.
- Barberry. Barberry can be used to treat gastrointestinal disorders and skin infections.

- Bilberry. This aids in improving blood circulation and repairs blood veins.
- Bitter orange. This is used to treat allergic inflammation.
- Blueberries. In addition to being a powerful antioxidants, they can be used to treat urinary tract infections.
- Cat's claw. This is used to treat gastrointestinal disorder, to boost the immune system and as an anti-inflammatory agent.
- Celery. This can be used as a diuretic.
- Chaste berry. This is used to treat PMS and menopausal symptoms and acne.
- Cilantro. Aids in detoxifying the body and in digestion.
- Clove. This can be ingested to treat an upset stomach and applied topically to treat toothaches.
- Cranberry. This aids in treating urinary tract infections.
- Daisy. These can be ingested as a tea, and the leaves can be used in a salad. It can be used to treat respiratory tract and gastrointestinal disorders.
- Devil's claw. This is used to treat back pain, joint inflammation, and arthritis.
- Dong Quai. This is used to treat the symptoms of PMS and menopause in addition to treating migraines and cardiovascular problems.
- Echinacea. The purple flowers of this plant aids in treating the common cold, helps to boost immunity, and treats bronchitis and upper respiratory infections.

- Evening primrose. This helps relieve the symptoms of PMS and menopause. It also aids in treating mild skin conditions such as eczema, helps to regulate blood pressure and is an anti-inflammatory.
- Eucalyptus. This can be used as an analgesic and to treat coughs and colds.
- Fenugreek. This can be used to treat the symptoms of menopause in addition to digestive issues and loss of appetite.
- Feverfew. Just as the name suggests, the leaves of this plant are used to treat fevers in addition to treating migraines and arthritis.
- Flaxseed. This is an anti-inflammatory, aids in weight loss management, aids in regulating blood pressure, and helps prevent colon cancer.
- Ginger. This aids in treating motion sickness and nausea.
- Gingko. This plant helps boost brain health and treats degenerative diseases like mild to moderate dementia and Alzheimer's disease. It also aids in treating mental illnesses, such as depression and anxiety and improving eye health.
- Ginseng. This can be used as an aphrodisiac and as a tonic to enhance vitality.
- Goldenseal. This is used to treat diarrhea, skin infections, and eye irritations. It can also be used as an antiseptic.
- Grape seed extract. This aids in lowering bad (LDL) cholesterol, regulating blood pressure, reducing the symptoms of poor circulation in leg veins, and is an anti-cancer agent.

- Green tea. The leaves of these can be used as a tonic to improve overall health and as an antioxidant.
- Guarana. This plant can be used as a tonic, to treat diarrhoea and control appetite.
- Guava. It can be used to treat diarrhea.
- Henna. This is an antibacterial and anti-inflammatory agent that has analgesic properties
- Horsetail. This can be used to treat tuberculosis and kidney problems in addition to healing wounds and ulcers and stopping bleeding.
- Jasmine. This is an anti-inflammatory and antiseptic agent.
- Lemon. The resulting liquid from combining the juice of this plant with honey can be used to treat sore throats and coughs.
- Milk thistle. The fruit of this plant is used to treat high cholesterol and liver condition in addition to reducing the growth of cancer cells.
- Mullein. Commonly added to cough syrups, this plant helps heal bronchial respiratory infections.
- Oregano. This can be used to treat stomach and respiratory ailments.
- Papaya. This can be used to treat stomach aches and wounds.
- Plantain. The leaves of this plant can be brewed in a tea, which can be used to fight coughs. The leaves can also be applied topically to treat skin infections and insect bites.

- Saint John's wort. The leaf and flower of this plant can be used as an antidepressant.
- Saw palmetto. The fruit of this plant can be used to treat benign prostatic hypertrophy.
- Star anise. This can be used to treat influenza.
- Tea tree oil. This oil is derived from the leaves of a tree that is native to Australia. It is beneficial in treating acne, dandruff, insect bites, and athlete's foot.
- Turmeric. This is an anti-inflammatory and aids in treating arthritis and skin diseases. It also aids in stopping the DNA mutations and helps prevent cancer.
- Valerian. The roots of this plant can be used to treat anxiety and as a sleep aid.
- Watercress. This can be used as an antibacterial agent and as a diuretic.
- Wild yam. This can be used to treat the symptoms of PMS and menopause in addition to being an anti-inflammatory agent. It also aids in relaxing muscles.

# Chapter 10: Medicinal Garden

You do not have to have a green thumb to grow an amazing medicinal herb and spice garden. This section is dedicated to showing you some of the easiest plants to grow and how you can maintain this garden no matter the amount of space that you have at your disposal. To relief from diarrhea and migraines and many other health issues, you can have them all by just stepping outside of your door. Keep reading to learn more.

## Benefits of Planting Your Own Medicinal Garden

There are several benefits to growing your own medicinal spice and herb garden. They include:

- Having more control over what you put into your body. Even though you pick up herbs and spices on your market or grocery store shelf, you have no way of truly knowing how these were grown and what chemicals that were used to assist the growth and maintenance process even if they claim to be organic. Chemicals like fertilizers can leave trace amounts on the plants, and these amounts can be ingested when we eat them. No matter how small these amounts are, they can burden us with dangerous their side effects and negative health consequences. By growing your own garden, you can have the security of knowing it is truly organic.

- Saving money. Often, all you need to get started with your own herb and spice garden is a packet of seeds. These cost next to nothing and keep on giving since the plants produce their own seeds most times. In addition, using these organic plants save you thousands of dollars in doctor's visits and bills every year when the resulting plants are used medicinally and in eating.

- Having a positive environmental impact. Gardens of all types attract insects like bees, butterflies and birds because they live off of the plants and the other types of creatures they attract. Birds and bees are pollinators and aid in ensuring more plants grow for the greater good of the earth.

- Gardening is good for your health. There are the obvious health benefits of eating organic plants from your own garden, like getting a greater variety of vitamins and minerals and lowering the risk of developing certain diseases. However, there are other health benefits, such as doing more physical activity that helps to keep your heart strong and taking in fresh air, which aids in purifying the lungs. There is also the mental health benefit of aiding in fighting mental diseases, such as depression.

- Gardening allows you to feel more self-reliant. When you have your own garden, you are not reliant on the supply from supermarkets or big corporations that make the big bucks off of your need to eat and to have good health. This aids in boosting your sense of independence and self-sufficiency.

- Gardening makes your yard more beautiful. Fruits, vegetables, flowers, herbs, and spices come in all sizes, shapes, and colors. These variations help to break up the monotonous nature of concrete jungles. The variety brings vivacity to the landscape and makes the scenery more interesting to look at. These plants also bring life ad beauty inside homes and offices.

- Garden helps bring you back to your indigenous roots. There is something about turning soil and planting seeds that makes a person feel more connected with the earth and to our ancestors who used to garden, not out of convenience, but out of necessity for medicine and food.

# Planning Your Garden

The reason most gardens fail is not because the person does not have a green thumb or because the process is particularly tricky. It is because these people begin to garden without any garden knowledge or planning. Here are some of the considerations you need to make to ensure that your medicinal garden flourishes:

- Your climate
- The location
- Choosing the right herbs and spices for your garden
- After care of your plants and herbs and spices

*The Types of Herbs and Spices That Should Be Planted in Different Climates*

Before you tried to plant any herb or spice in your garden, you need to ensure that the temperature range of the climate that you live in is suitable for growing that particular plant. A little research on the Internet or speaking with your local nursery can help you with this. Summer and tropical climates are great for growing most plants. However, winter type climates are less forgiving.

## Plants That Grow Well in Warm and Hot Climates

All of the burbs and spices that will be listed below require that the soil be well-drained and need to be attended to when conditions are soggy. Some plants need to be planted at the required distance apart so that they are not crowded and air circulation is not compromised.

The following plants need at least four hours of bright sunlight per day and thrive in morning sunlight. They include parsley, peppermint, rosemary, sage, tarragon, mint, oregano, cilantro, basil, and chives.

These plants need between six and eight hours of direct sunlight daily. They include dill, fennel, yarrow, licorice, lavender, and winter savory.

## Plants That Grow Well in Cold Climates

While winter has fewer hours of sunlight and the chilling temperature can make it harder to grow herbs and spices, it is not impossible to do especially if you have an indoor garden or if you can temporarily house the plants inside. Many of the herbs and spices listed can be grown year-round as long as the proper care and precaution is taken to ensure that they still thrive during the winter months. Some of them go dormant in the winter months and come back with new growth in the spring.

To prepare these plants for winter, prune them a few weeks before the first frost of the fall season by removing any wooden or dead stems and snipping off the upper leaves. This will ensure that your plant has a better chance of surviving from winter to spring.

You can still use some of these plants throughout the winter by digging them up and transferring them to containers that will be kept indoors by a sunny window throughout the winter. Out of some of the herbs and spices listed above that grow great in warm and hot climates, there are a few that can also survive the winter weather as long as they are kept indoors next to a sunny window. They include oregano, sage, mint, chives, and thyme. On the other hand, there are herbs and spices that are well adapted to growing in cold weather and they include tarragon, lemon balm, catnip, parsley, horseradish, sorrel, and caraway.

## *Choosing the Right Location*

When choosing a location to grow your medicinal garden, the two factors you need to consider are how well lit the area is by sunlight and the availability of well-drained soil. Therefore, you can grow your medicinal garden if you have acres of yard space available or even if you live in a tiny apartment.

No matter what location you choose or have available for your garden, here are a few tips to get you started, especially if this is your first time trying your hand at gardening:

- Start small. This tip is especially useful if you live in an apartment or do not have much space for a garden. If you have yard space available, cultivate your plants in a few feet of space to see how it goes. If you live in an apartment, get one or two small pots. Herbs and spices like basil, chives, geranium, thyme, parsley, mint, bay laurel, and rosemary are great for planting in small spaces or in an apartment.

- Focus on growing a few different plants to begin with. Do not overdo it or try to grow every herb or spice that you can think of. Start with herbs and spices that you already use regularly and are relatively easy to grow.

- Choose an area that receives adequate sunlight or is lit by natural light bulbs to place your potted plants or to cultivate your yard space.

- Research the plants that you plan to plant so that you know that the conditions it thrives and avoid placing it under conditions that will destroy it.

- Use good soil to get started. Different plants need different types of soil to grow. Usually herbs and spices grow best in typical garden soil because it has good drainage. Most herbs and spices do not do well in sandy soil or heavy clay so adding compost can be a good option if these are the types of soil that you have available. Compost provides the soil with needed nutrition to help plants grow.

- Get a few worms. Worms do a great job at breaking down the organics in soil, which makes them easier for plants to absorb. Worms can usually be purchased at bait and tackle shops.

- Set a watering schedule for your plants. Some plants need to be watered more often than others. Over-watering can damage a plant as can under-watering. Research will tell you how much your plants need to be watered so that you can set up a proper schedule to keep the plants properly hydrated.

- Learn how to weed. Luckily, this is not a concern if you live in an apartment, but if you have yard space then you need to set up a schedule for this as well.

- Keep it interesting. As you get your footing with gardening, gradually add new plants to your collection and have fun with it.

# 9 Common Herbs and Spices That You Can Grow on Your Own

## *Rosemary*

Rosemary is an evergreen shrub that produces blue flowers and has needle-like leaves. The scientific name of rosemary is rosmarinus officinalis. This scientific name translates into "mists of the seas" because of its gray-green color, which resembles the mist against the cliff of the seaside of the Mediterranean, where the plant originates.

The health benefits of rosemary include levels of antioxidants, acting as an anti-inflammatory, improving digestion, preventing brain aging, lowering the risk of developing certain cancers, and enhancing memory and concentration.

Rosemary is not a plant that is complicated to care for. All it needs is well-drained, sandy soil and between six and eight hours of sunlight. It thrives in warm, humid environments and cannot withstand temperatures below 50 degrees Fahrenheit. Therefore, it needs to be transplanted from the soil to a container during winter months and kept indoors near a sunny window.

Rosemary plants are usually grown via the cuttings because the seeds are tricky to germinate. In fact, the seeds only germinate when they are very fresh and planted in conditions that are optimum. To propagate rosemary plants using cuttings, cut a two-inch stem from an existing to rosemary plant and remove the leaves on the bottom two-thirds of the way down of the cutting. Place this cutting in a mixture of peat moss and pertile. Spray the cutting with water. Once the roots have developed, the plants should successfully grow. Rosemary plants should be repotted at least once every year because they have a tendency to become root bound, which is the condition that causes a plant's roots to fill its container, leaving no more room for the plant to expand. Luckily, the yellowing of the plant will indicate that it is time to repot.

## *Parsley*

Parsley comes from the same family as dill and has bright green, feather-like leaves. It is a biennial plant, which means that it takes two years to complete its life cycle. During the first year, its leaves, stems and roots grow, then it enters a period of dormancy in the winter months. Next, the plant flowers and produces fruits and seeds before it dies.

Parsley can be used to make soups, salads, and sauces in addition to being a garnish. It is often used in detoxing juice cleanses and medicinally to reduce the risk of developing certain cancers, improve the function of the immune system, reduce inflammation, protect the blood vessels, and reduce the risk of developing diseases such as type 2 diabetes and asthma.

To plant parsley, individual seeds need to be placed in pots indoors for 10 to 12 weeks before the last spring frost. Soaking the seeds overnight before planting makes for better germination. The seeds should be planted in moist, rich soil with six to eight inches between them. The soil should be around 70 degrees Fahrenheit for best growth. Placing a fluorescent light above the seedlings makes them grow faster and healthier. When planting parsley, it is best to place them near tomatoes, corn, and asparagus in your garden. Continue to water the seeds daily so that they do not dry out during the process of germination.

Parsley is ready to be harvested when the leaf stems have three segments. The leaves from the outer portions can be cut, but the inner portions should be left on the plant to mature. Parsley can be stored by placing the stalk in water and keeping refrigerated or in dry storage by cutting the base of the parsley and hanging them in a well-ventilated warm and shady area. Once the parsley has completely dried, crumble it and store in an airtight container. You can enjoy parsley throughout the winter by replanting the parsley plant in a container and keeping it near a sunny window indoors.

### *Thyme*

This herb is used to make soups, grilled meat, and vegetables taste wonderful. It is a fragrant herb that has small leaves and a thin wooden stem. It comes in over 50 varieties and originated from the Mediterranean. Its health benefits include lowering blood pressure, boosting immunity, being a cough suppressant, being an insect repellent and a mood booster.

Thyme is an herb that loves heat and grows best in temperatures of around 70 degrees Fahrenheit. The soil needs to be well-drained. It is easiest to grow thyme from the plant cuttings around two to three weeks before the last spring frost. Plant the cuttings about nine inches apart. Thyme should be grown next to tomatoes and cabbages in your garden. Just like rosemary, this can be transplanted to a container in the winter months and left next to a sunny window to grow.

This plant should be watered deeply only when the soil has completely dried out. It should be pruned in the spring and summer months to contain its growth. This plant needs to be replaced when they are about three to four years old because the leaves become less flavorful and the stem becomes woodier.

Thyme can be harvested by cutting about five inches of growth while leaving the lower your parts behind. It is best to harvest thyme in the morning before the dew has dried out. Thyme should be stored and refrigerated for one to two weeks while lightly packaged in plastic. For drying thyme, hang the sprigs in a well-ventilated, warm and dry area. When the spring have dried out, crush them and store in an airtight container for up to two years.

### *Mint*

This herb has a fruity aromatic taste and flowers pink, purple, and white buds. This plant has several varieties. This plant spreads very easily so you need to be careful where you plant it. Mint thrives in well-drained soil and may require some protection from direct sunlight. When mint is grown indoors, it is best to grow it in a confined area such as a container, especially since they needed protection in the colder months of winter. Plant mint next to tomatoes and cabbages in a garden.

Mint is propagated by using cuttings that are about six inches long. These need to be placed horizontally in the soil or placed to root in a glass of water.

Mint does not require much care. When it is planted outdoors, use light mulch to keep the soil moist and the leaves clean. When it is planted indoors, it needs to be watered regularly to keep the soil moist.

Mint needs to be harvested frequently due to its penchant for overgrowth and because young leaves have more flavor than older ones. Mint can be harvested as soon as it pops up in spring. Mint can be stored frozen or air-dried.

### Basil

Basil is great for bring flavor to soups, smoothies, juices, Italian dishes, pesto, and as a garnish. This plant thrives in warm weather. The most common types of basil are sweet basil, purple basil, lemon basil, and Thai basil. Even though basil is easy to grow and maintain, it should only be grown outdoors in summer. Ideally, it should be planted six weeks before the last spring frost and after the well-drained but moist soil has warmed up to at least 70 degrees Fahrenheit. Nighttime temperature should not go below 50 degrees Fahrenheit. The plant also needs to be planted in an area that gets between six and eight hours of sunlight daily. Without this heat, the plant will not grow.

To plant basil, the seeds should be placed about ¼-inch deep into the soil with about 12 inches placed between. Basil grow best when planted next to tomatoes.

After the bud has produced at least six leaves, prune the plant to about the second set to encourage branching. This encourages the growth of more leaves for harvesting. Repeat this pruning process every time that the basil produced their first set of leaves. Pinch off the center six-weeks after germination to prevent early flowering. If flowers grow, cut them off.

If the weather suddenly becomes cold, harvest the plant because the chilly weather will destroy it.

## *Winter Savory*

The scientific name of winter savory is satureja montana. It is an annual plant and has a strong, peppery flavor. The plant has dark green, glossy leaves, and woody stems. It grows best when exposed to at least six hours of sunlight daily and when planted in well-drained soil that has a pH of 6.7. The seeds should be planted in spring outdoors in pots and transplanted to a garden about 10 inches apart. Winter savory can also be propagated through cuttings in late spring. The cuttings should be placed in pots filled with wet sand. The sprouts can then be transplanted to a container or garden. This plant will become dormant in the winter months and will put out new leaves in spring. Pruning encourages new growth. The health benefits of this plant include treating diarrhea and nausea, treating sore throats, as a tonic, as a cough suppressant and to increase sex drive.

This planted can be used to make essential oils. The leaves can also be used fresh or dried.

## *Oregano*

This plant can be used to fight bacterial infections, for its anti-cancer properties, for its antioxidant properties, to reduce viral infections, and to decrease inflammation. This herb has a taste that is similar to thyme and can be used in a variety of tasty dishes. It is commonly used in Italian dishes.

This is a plant that loves warm weather, and it is usually planted late in the spring season. It can be propagated from seeds or cuttings between 6 and 10 weeks before the last spring frost. Either seeds or cuttings can be placed in well-drained soil that has a temperature of around 70 degrees Fahrenheit. Plants should be planted at least 10 inches apart and can be planted next to any vegetable or herb in your garden.

To care for oregano plants, allow them to grow to about four-inches tall and then trim to encourage branching and higher leaf density. Oregano is a plant that does not require much care and does not need to be watered as often as most herbs. Water the oregano when the soil feels dry.

Leaves can be harvested as needed and the most flavorful ones are found right before the plant blooms flowers. Oregon leaves can be stored by freezing and air drying them. Once they are dried, keep them stored in an airtight container.

### *Sage*

Sage, whose scientific name is salvia officinalis, is a plant that is easy to grow and adds a lot of flavor to dishes, especially meats and bean dishes. The leaves of the sage plant are gray-green in color and its flowers can be blue, pink, white, and purple.

Sage will not grow in wet soil; therefore, should be planted in well-drained soil. The best and easiest way to propagate sage is from a small plant. Seeds can also be planted two weeks before the last spring frost. Cuttings can be planted one or two weeks before the last spring frost.

Soil temperature should be between 60 and 70 degrees Fahrenheit, and plants should be grown in close proximity to rosemary, cabbage and carrots in a garden. Keep them far away from cucumbers.

To care for sage, the young plants should be watered regularly so that they grow quickly at which point watering can be decreased. It is best to replace these plants every few years. They should be pruned every spring.

To harvest sage, harvest lightly during the first year of growth by pinching off the leaves or by snipping off small sprigs from the plant. Once the first year has passed, you only need to leave a few stalks so that the plants can rejuvenate in the future. Once the plant has fully established itself, it can be harvested up to three times in one season. Do not harvest the plant in the fall so that it can prepare for winter. Sage can be stored by freezing or drying, it but can be used fresh as well.

The health benefits of sage include being an antioxidant, supporting good oral health, easing the symptoms of menopause, reducing blood sugar levels, supporting brain health, lowering bad cholesterol levels, protecting against certain cancers, alleviating diarrhea and supporting bone health.

## *Sorrel*

Sorel is an herb with a tangy, lemony flavor. The flowers are commonly used to make juices. The sorrel leaves can be steamed or sautéed just as you would spinach. They can also be used in salads, soups, and sauces. The leaves are commonly used in French cuisine. There are several varieties of sorrel, but they are all known for the health benefits of lowering blood pressure, decreasing bad cholesterol levels, detoxifying the body and as an antioxidant.

Sorrel grows in temperate conditions in damp soil in open areas. Sorrel can be sown from the seeds or by dividing the roots. The best time to propagate sorrel is in June or July. The flowers bloom quickly after and can be used to make juice. This slows down the production of leaves so if you want more leaf production, cut off the flower stalks. Cutting off the flower stalks also gives you more harvests. You can cut the plant to the ground and it will produce a new crop.

Sorrel can be harvested late in the spring until fall or when the plant is about six inches tall. Both the flower and the leaves can be harvested.

# Conclusion

Billions of dollars are exchanged every year for the human race to obtain healthcare. Every year the amount spent increases because every year pharmaceutical companies find new ways of ensuring we are tricked into thinking that they are dependent on prescription drugs to make living bearable. We have been duped into believing that life cannot no longer be a fun, enjoyable, healthy adventure because sickness is spreading like wildfire and this is all part of the propaganda designed by these big name companies.

It is a sad truth that human disease and illness is a big business for the pharmaceutical companies and doctors. These are the people we have placed our faith in to keep us healthy but that trust is being broken because pharmaceutical drugs come with a host of side effects that can make us even more unwell than when they started the use of pharmaceutical drugs. Even more unfortunate is the fact that these side effects are considered mild most times. How can they possibly be mild when they disrupt our daily lives and lower the quality of the way we live? How can being a diarrhea or suffering from dizziness or nausea be considered mild when you cannot leave the house for fear that these side effects will embarrass you or place your life in danger?

And what of the more 'serious' side effects like internal bleeding, liver damage, and heart disease that are whispered in commercials like the inconsequential? But these side effects are far from inconsequential. They matter just as your health and wellness does. And it is an insult us that pharmaceutical downplay the severity of these side effects.

It is time that we stopped being slaves to pharmaceutical companies and doctors that use our pain for their gain. There is a better way to obtain the good health that you desire, and it comes free of charge most often. Human health is the most valuable resource that we will ever own and it is about time that it be treated with the high worth that it has.

## Plant-Based Medicine Worked for Our Ancestors and It Can Work for You Too

Before the invention of technology and money, our ancestors took to the earth and planted herbs and spices that they used to treat illnesses that range from mild to serious. There was no monopoly of resources or manipulation for profit. Our ancestors simply when outside and pick a plant from the garden to find a cure for an illness and to prevent the development of a disease. This seems like a lost time, but it does not have to be. You too can benefit from naturally grown medications instead of risking your health with synthetics.

## Plant-Based Eating Can Change Your Life for the Better

Plants not only provide us with powerful medicinal effects but they also provide us with powerful nutrition, detoxification, and other health benefits such as improved function of the immune system and lowered risk of developing several other diseases such as obesity, cardiovascular disease, digestive issues, and mental illness. The powerful compounds in plants are so effective that pharmaceutical companies try to imitate the effects. But nothing beats the natural way.

## Take Control of Your Overall Health

The pages of this book are packed with powerful information that allows you to take control of not only your health but your entire life because they not only contain information on medicinal practices but how to improve your eating habits and detoxify your body. There is nothing stopping you from being the healthier, happier, and more productive individual that you can be. It is possible to cure and prevent illnesses without suffering from side effects. It is possible to eat healthier without having to drive through a restaurant that serves questionable ingredients and buy ingredients that are filled with the remnants of fertilizers. It is possible to get rid of the toxins that modern pollution and bad eating habits have made common in the human body. It is possible to make your immune system stronger than ever by fortifying it with nutrition and probiotics.

All of this and more are possible by stepping out into your yard or plucking a leaf from your kitchen garden. You can control your health to such an extent that you do not even have to go to the grocery store to stock up on healthy eating and medicinal ingredients. You can get it all right there in your own garden even if you live in a small space.

## *A Final Word*

We all want to live healthier lives. Being in good health makes us happier, less stressed, and makes life feel like it is worth living. Being sick can drain us and make life seem hopeless, especially when you have been prescribed pill after pill and tablet upon tablet and you are seeing little to no results. This kind of life is no better than living as a slave and, in this case, it is being a slave to pharmaceutical corporations that bank on you never fully recovering. Fortunately, you can break free of the shackles at any time on any day. Taking a plant-based approach to medicine and eating places you as the one in control of your life, which is the way that it should.

This book was written with careful consideration and packed with tons of knowledge to place you well on your way to living a life that is healthier and therefore, happier. I hope that the tips outlined have been solidified in your mind so that you can start acting today. None of these tips will do any good if you do not get proactive. You need to take action to see the results. If you need to, do not be afraid to go back and read the particular sections that are of interest to you. While you at it, share this book with a friend or family member so that they too can break free of the shackles that pharmaceutical companies have imprisoned us with.

# References

Bent S. (2008). Herbal medicine in the United States: a review of efficacy, safety, and regulation: grand rounds at the University of California, San Francisco Medical Center. *Journal of general internal medicine, 23*(6), 854–859. doi:10.1007/s11606-008-0632-y

DeAngelis C. D. (2016). Big Pharma Profits and the Public Loses. *The Milbank quarterly, 94*(1), 30–33. doi:10.1111/1468-0009.12171

Ferner R. E. (2005). The influence of big pharma. *BMJ (Clinical research ed.), 330*(7496), 855–856. doi:10.1136/bmj.330.7496.855

Firenzuoli, F., & Gori, L. (2007). Herbal medicine today: clinical and research issues. *Evidence-based complementary and alternative medicine : eCAM, 4*(Suppl 1), 37–40. doi:10.1093/ecam/nem096

Hajar R. (2012). The air of history: early medicine to galen (part I). *Heart views : the official journal of the Gulf Heart Association, 13*(3), 120–128. doi:10.4103/1995-705X.102164

Nicholson L. B. (2016). The immune system. *Essays in biochemistry, 60*(3), 275–301. doi:10.1042/EBC20160017

Ostfeld R. J. (2017). Definition of a plant-based diet and overview of this special issue. *Journal of geriatric cardiology : JGC, 14*(5), 315. doi:10.11909/j.issn.1671-5411.2017.05.008

Rang H. (2013). Bad Pharma: how drug companies mislead doctors and harm patients. *British Journal of Clinical Pharmacology, 75*(5), 1377–1379. doi:10.1111/bcp.12047

Welz, A. N., Emberger-Klein, A., & Menrad, K. (2018). Why people use herbal medicine: insights from a focus-group study in Germany. *BMC complementary and alternative medicine, 18*(1), 92. doi:10.1186/s12906-018-2160-6

Made in the USA
Columbia, SC
16 May 2020